P9-DWI-798

Advance Praise for Kimberly Snyder and *The Beauty Detox Solution*

"I don't like to diet, I like to eat right and that's what Kim's philosophy is all about. Her food program has had such an impact not only on my body but also on my health in general. She's brilliant."

—Drew Barrymore

"Kimberly Snyder's *The Beauty Detox Solution* is a must-read that intelligently highlights the importance of incorporating large amounts of greens and plant foods into our diet. It also provides the reader with innovative ways to maximize their consumption."

—Dr. Mehmet Oz
Coauthor of the YOU book series

"I was introduced to Kimberly and her Glowing Green Smoothie and it's now the staple of my daily regimen that I won't skip. When it comes to health and nutrition, Kimberly is a real expert and her nutritional concepts are easy to follow, make sense and will increase your energy and vitality. After reading this book there really isn't an excuse not to be healthy."

—Owen Wilson

"Experiencing Kimberly's food on set is what made me want to read *The Beauty Detox Solution*. It tastes so great, it changed the way I viewed living foods. It isn't all nuts and oils! I really enjoyed reading this book and it's packed with so much great information. Most important, her food program will appeal to everyone and take away the fear associated with a greens based diet."

—Olivia Wilde

"Kimberly is beyond beautiful. Her healthy Banana Fro-Yo recipe is amazing, delicious and you would never know that it's not frozen yogurt."

—Jillian Barbarie
Host, *Good Day LA*

"Kimberly is my go-to for health and nutrition. Her nutritional concepts have made a really big difference in the way I feel. They allow you to enjoy food that tastes great, but is also healthy and makes you feel fantastic all day long."

—Justin Long

"When I began Kimberly Snyder's program I began to see results immediately. I lost the unwanted pounds and felt much more mentally focused. Kimberly gives you the knowledge and tools to look and feel your best the natural way."

—Jeff Lewis
Star of Bravo's hit TV show *Flipping Out*

"When you're working long hours on a movie set, it can be exhausting. On my last film, I was introduced to Kimberly and her amazing Glowing Green Smoothie. I drank it every day and I love the way it tastes and how it gives me a burst of energy, while keeping me full and satisfied between meals. Kimberly's knowledge of health and nutrition is remarkable and her passionate energy on the subject is so contagious that it truly inspires you to be healthy."

—Peter Farrelly
Director, *There's Something About Mary* and *Dumb and Dumber*

"Kimberly is one of our all-time favorite nutritional experts. Her in-depth knowledge of nutrition, health and beauty is truly inspiring. We always get great feedback and responses whenever she is on the show, which is why she has an open invitation to come on the show anytime she is in Los Angeles."

—Michelle Pulfrey
Producer, *Good Day LA*

"Kim Snyder's book, *The Beauty Detox Solution,* combines modern concepts of dietary detoxification with her worldwide experience and portfolio of recipes to show readers how to restore their body to its natural healthy state."

—John E. Strobeck, M.D., Ph.D.
Heart-Lung Center, Hawthorne, NJ

THE
BEAUTY
DETOX
SOLUTION

Eat Your Way to Radiant Skin, Renewed Energy
and the Body You've Always Wanted

KIMBERLY SNYDER, C.N.

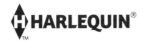

THE BEAUTY **DETOX** SOLUTION
ISBN-13: 978-0-373-89232-7
© 2011 by Kimberly Snyder
Illustrations by Curt Altmann.

All rights reserved. The reproduction, transmission or utilization of this work in whole or in part in any form by any electronic, mechanical or other means, now known or hereafter invented, including xerography, photocopying and recording, or in any information storage or retrieval system, is forbidden without the written permission of the publisher. For permission please contact Harlequin Enterprises, Ltd., 225 Duncan Mill Road, Don Mills, Ontario, Canada, M3B 3K9.

The health advice presented in this book is intended only as an informative resource guide to help you make informed decisions; it is not meant to replace the advice of a physician or to serve as a guide to self-treatment. Always seek competent medical help for any health condition or if there is any question about the appropriateness of a procedure or health recommendation.

Library of Congress Cataloging-in-Publication Data
Snyder, Kimberly.

The beauty detox solution : eat your way to radiant skin, renewed energy and the body you've always wanted / Kimberly Snyder.

p. cm.
Includes bibliographical references and index.

ISBN 978-0-373-89232-7 (pbk.)
1. Detoxification (Health) 2. Beauty, Personal. 3. Self-care, Health. I. Title.
RA784.5S69 2011
613—dc22
2010034169

® and TM are trademarks owned and used by the trademark owner and/or its licensee. Trademarks indicated with ® are registered in the United States Patent and Trademark Office, the Canadian Trade Marks Office and/or other countries.

www.eHarlequin.com

Printed in U.S.A.

This book is dedicated to you, my dear reader.

It is my sincere intention in writing this book to help you achieve your ultimate beauty and health. When we are free from constant worry about our physical appearance, we can direct our unlimited power toward accomplishing all of our personal, professional and spiritual goals.

I hope that applying this knowledge will free you, in the way it has freed me.

Cast away all negative thoughts and fears. If your will is yoked to wisdom, you can achieve anything.

—Paramahansa Yogananda

CONTENTS

Introduction   xi

PART 1: BEAUTY DETOX BASICS

Chapter 1: **Our Diet, Dictated by Nature**   1
How Our Body Is Designed   2
How Our Design Affects Our Diet   3
The Science Behind the Beauty Detox Solution   7
Cancer Risk   8
Heart Disease   9
Diabetes   10

Chapter 2: **Beauty Energy**   15
The Real Cause of Aging   17
A Clean Body Is a Beautiful Body   18
The Alkaline-Acid Principle   23
The 80-20 Ratio   27
The Beauty Food Circle   28

Chapter 3: **Eating for Beauty**   31
Eat Alkaline First   32
No More Calorie Counting   33
Beauty Food Pairing   36
How Beauty Food Pairing Works   39
Eat Light to Heavy   51
Speed Is Possible Only if We Avoid a Traffic Jam   51
Your Beauty Food Plan   54

Chapter 4: **Beauty Minerals and Enzymes**   65
Essential Beauty Minerals   67
Enzymes Build Beauty   67
Where Cooked Food Fits In   75
Minerals + Enzymes = Green Drinks   75

Chapter 5: **Beauty Foods**   83
Plant Protein Is Beauty Protein   84
There Is Nothing Beautiful About Dairy   99
Beautiful Carbohydrates and Starches   105
Choose Beauty Fats and Eat in Moderation   112
Fruit: The Ultimate Beauty Food   117
Beauty Greens and Vegetables   120

PART 2: YOUR BEAUTY SOLUTION

Chapter 6: **Detoxing for Beauty**   131
  Beauty Detox Secret #1: Probiotics   137
  Beauty Detox Secret #2: Plant-Based Digestive Enzymes   139
  Beauty Detox Secret #3: Probiotic & Enzyme Salad   140
  Beauty Detox Secret #4: Magnesium-Oxygen Supplement   143
  Beauty Detox Secret #5: Gravity-Centered Colonics and Enemas   144

Chapter 7: **Becoming Beautiful**   149
  The Importance of Transitioning   150
  The Beauty Phases   153
  Beauty Detox Portion Guidelines   159
  Your Beauty Detox Kitchen   160
  Your Beauty Detox Shopping List   163

Chapter 8: **Phase 1: Blossoming Beauty**   167
  Blossoming Beauty Benefits   168
  Blossoming Beauty Basic Tenets   169
  Blossoming Beauty Sample One-Week Menu   170

Chapter 9: **Phase 2: Radiant Beauty**   175
  Radiant Beauty Benefits   177
  Radiant Beauty Basic Tenets   177
  Radiant Beauty Sample One-Week Menu   179

Chapter 10: **Phase 3: True Beauty**   185
  True Beauty Benefits   186
  True Beauty Basic Tenets   186
  True Beauty Sample One-Week Menu   188

Chapter 11: **Beauty Recipes**   193
  The Everyday Beauty Basics   197
  Beauty Dips and Dressings   200
  Beauty Salads   207
  Beauty Wraps and Sandwiches   211
  Beauty Soups and Veggie Dishes   213
  Beauty Grain Dishes   217
  Beauty Nut Dishes   222
  Beauty Smoothies   226
  Beauty Desserts   228

Converting to Metric   231

Endnotes   232

Acknowledgments   237

Live the Beauty Detox Lifestyle   239

Index   241

About the Author   247

INTRODUCTION

Dearest Friend and Reader,

Welcome! I am just *thrilled* and honored that I get to share this journey with you as you discover your highest level of beauty and health.

I know how confusing it can be to navigate the numerous conflicting and ever-changing health philosophies that are out there. *Fruit is healthy. No, fruit has too much sugar! Be sure to count fat grams. No, wait. Make that to count carbs!* The conflicting advice used to always make me wonder if I was doing something wrong. What are we supposed to believe, and where do we turn for the answers?

Well, it *really* doesn't have to be that complicated. The goal of my book is to show you fundamental principles that will teach you how to unlock your highest potential beauty and achieve optimal health. As you'll find, it is actually very simple. And in our ever-progressing, complicated world, simplicity is a beautiful thing. We need not get swept up in the chaos of gimmicky new diets and worry if we are missing out on the Holy Grail of instant weight loss and wrinkle freedom. The truth is, it doesn't exist in the hot new diet. But there is an answer, and the exciting news is that it is right in front of you.

I want you to know right off the bat that this book is *not* about restriction in any sense. We will not be counting calories or grams of carbs, and we will not be restricted to eating in one particular way to fit into one dietary category. You can discover your ultimate health and beauty whether you are a vegan, vegetarian, raw foodist, pescatarian or omnivore. The broad concepts I outline in this book will work for everyone, and you will see and feel results, whatever your current diet. There is a phase, or eating plan, that works for everyone—regardless of lifestyle, budget or personal tastes.

Once we get rid of restriction and embrace the idea of consuming an *abundance* of the right foods, we free ourselves up to understand, internalize and apply the true tenets of health and beauty. With just a few simple changes, you will look and feel better than you ever have before. That is my promise to you!

And the best part? You'll have all these benefits without counting calories or obsessing over tiny portion sizes or eating bland microwaved foods! You will be feasting on fresh, delicious and filling foods that will nourish every cell in your body so that a deeply healthful, radiant glow permeates from within. Your skin will become brighter, your hair shinier and your body more toned. Belly fat will drop off, and your eyes will sparkle with newfound energy. You can achieve true health and beauty naturally with *food.* This diet is that powerful.

I believe the word "health" is synonymous with the word "beauty." A healthy body is a beautiful body. Healthy skin, which is a reflection of our internal health, is beautiful skin. My definition of beauty is that it should be deep, lasting and magnetic, and grow from the inside out. The key to this kind of vibrant beauty is ongoing cleansing. When your cells and blood are clean and detoxified, your body is able to function optimally and you are able to maximize the use of plentiful minerals in your food. Your skin will radiate from the inside out, excess pounds will melt away and your body will achieve its perfect weight. We've all seen the kind of beauty I'm talking about. A woman who just *glows.* Now you, too, can sparkle with true beauty.

I wrote this book to help free you from wasting time and energy struggling with debilitating new diets and cleanses, wearing layers and layers of concealer and foundation to hide dulled, flawed skin and, yes, squeezing into your "fat" jeans. I promise you that it *is* possible to achieve your most beautiful self and your perfect weight—while eating abundantly! And once you stop wasting time and energy worrying about your skin and weight, you can focus on your real goals and dreams.

Believe me, I have had my own share of weight and beauty battles. I struggled for years to control my weight as a superthin, calorie- and fat-gram-counting marathon runner. I was always swallowing a gnawing hunger, and at five foot five I was barely one hundred pounds, with hair as coarse as steel wool. Then I went in the totally opposite direction (yes, I admit it!). After graduating from college, I moved to Sydney, Australia, where I landed my first job. For my job, I was mingling with the A-list celebrity crowd, riding yachts and constantly eating out at fancy dinners and, yes, drinking expensive wine and partying.

I was spending all my time involved in activities I thought were so glamorous. *Hey, you're relaxing,* I told myself. *Have another glass.* Well, what I thought was healthy food—soy burgers, fat-free milk, pretzels, yogurt, sushi and grilled veggie and mozzarella sandwiches—added over thirty pounds to my small frame! My skin was a dull, zit-covered mess, and I believe that I looked older than I do now. I stopped working out regularly because I just didn't have the energy. Instead I turned to soy milk cappuccinos and Diet Coke to give me periodic "boosts" throughout the day.

When I developed a roll of fat on my once flat-as-a-board belly, I looked in the mirror and decided that I couldn't take it anymore. It was at that point that a new and highly influential person came into my life: an Australian holistic nutritionist who ran a nutritional detox center in Sydney. By chance (since I went so infrequently) I saw a small flyer of hers at the gym.

I had never before tried to do anything remotely detox related, but I was desperate for something to help and decided to give it a shot. This gorgeous, blond forty-something-year-old with sharp green eyes assessed my bumpy skin, my dull hair and the ridges in my nails and gave me a knowing look. She shook her head when she saw the thick coating of mucus on my tongue. The first questions she asked me were, "How often do you go to the bathroom?" and "Do you get bloated and gassy often?"

To which I replied, "What? Who cares about *that* stuff? I want to lose weight and make my skin look better!"

She smiled. "*That* stuff is what it is all about, my dear."

I was put on a stern detox program, cutting out dairy and refined carbs, like pretzels and white rice, from my diet immediately. This Aussie guru also made me concoctions for my liver with nineteen medicinal plants, my first introduction to the bounty of herbs in Ayurvedic and Chinese medicine. She also made her own face and body creams, and she forever changed the way I thought about my skin. She helped me see that the skin is our largest organ and functions like a mirror of what's going on inside the body: it offers us a direct reflection of the health achievements we make and the obstacles with which we struggle. My skin held all the answers, and all I had to do was pay attention to what it was telling me. Likewise, I learned that from 60 to 70 percent of what we put on our skin is absorbed through the skin into our bloodstream and liver. That certainly changed the way I thought of beauty products for good!

She jolted something awake in me and inspired my voracious passion for both natural health and skin care. I stopped partying and going out to dinner parties every night and read all the information and books the nutritionist gave me. I spent a lot of time with her, shopping at health stores, sipping herbal tea, and walking along Bondi Beach, where we both lived, having health discussions for hours. We became very close friends! The more I followed her advice, the better I looked and felt. The weight I'd gained melted off, and my skin started to clear up. I had so much energy that any thought of "needing" a coffee got banished from my mind! The results were incredible.

I knew I had to make a complete break from my current path in life. I didn't want to simply change the way I ate; I wanted to profoundly change the way I lived. Learning about natural health and skin care and the natural healing properties of plants made me jittery inside. I was so excited! Even though I still had no idea how this new interest would fit into my life, I was thrilled about the unknown possibilities. I could no longer ignore the dull ache in my heart telling me that I was on the wrong career path, in a corporate field that was not my real passion. I had found something I was incredibly passionate about: learning more and more about how food itself is medicine and a powerful tool for achieving our highest beauty.

Once I came to realize what I truly wanted, the flame was lit and inspiration shifted into action. I was in a serious long-distance relationship with someone back home, but I knew deep down that it wasn't right. Within one week I quit my job, declined law school for the following fall, broke my apartment lease on Bondi Beach and dumped my boyfriend. There was no turning back now!

I walked into an STA travel office and, with a few thousand dollars saved from working, bought an around-the-world ticket with fifteen stops across five continents. At first I thought I might travel for two or three weeks, but once I started out, I could not stop. The more I learned and saw, the more I wanted to explore... so I ended up traveling for a total of about three years to very remote communities, for dollars a day. I stayed in guesthouses, ashrams, my tent (for many months across Africa), bungalows, on floors (even a few times on the floors of Asian Laundromats), and sometimes in bus and train stations with my backpack strapped to my body. I started out alone but sporadically met up with old friends and constantly met new people along the way as I weaved my way through Laos, China,

Mongolia, Nepal, India, Swaziland, Indonesia, New Zealand, Cambodia, Mozambique, Zimbabwe, Croatia, Peru, Malaysia, Botswana...over fifty countries in all.

My adventures were at times rough, dirty and even dangerous (though nothing really bad ever happened), but the truth is that I gleaned an incredible education from my three-year around-the-world journey. All these diverse countries had one thing in common: they had their own secrets to health and beauty. Each had an impact on my perspective on health, and in each country I deepened my understanding of true beauty and learned powerful beauty tips I still treasure today.

Thailand was the first country I ventured to after I left Australia, and it marked my initial immersion in the wonderful world of ancient and beautifying Asian fruits, especially the legendary durian. I feasted on the abundance of local fruit, and it composed a good 70 percent of my diet. It was then that I began my lifelong obsession with young coconuts, eating them every day, and like many Thais, I began using coconut oil on my hair and my body. Acquainting myself with all the culturally important fruits made me feel closely connected to the earth there, as well as to the warm, friendly and deeply Buddhist Thai people. When I came back to the United States, I continued to study coconuts and discovered that coconut oil is amazingly beautifying: it is cholesterol free and rich in medium-chain good fats that nourish the skin.

Hunan Province, tucked away in southwest China and home to many hill-tribe villages, is another one of my favorite parts of the world. I spent several weeks bicycling across rice paddies and sleeping on the floor of rooms in guesthouses, covered by mosquito nets. I noticed that the women with beautiful, glowing skin there consumed goji berries, no dairy, very small portions of meat and lots of local vegetables. I became fascinated with the depth of natural health knowledge so prevalent in China's culture, including its focus on ancient medicinal herbs and ways to enhance the chi (or life force) of the body by treating it as a holistic unit, rather than treating only one organ at a time.

My time in the Himalayas, which included months in Nepal, Kashmir and other parts of northern India, was simply magical. It was there that I first discovered yoga, which would have a lifelong impact on me. I also enjoyed greater exposure to Ayurvedic teachings and, in particular, became fascinated with the spice turmeric, which was first given to me by a tiny elderly woman as wrinkled as a raisin who ran an Ayurvedic healing center in a mountain nook. The turmeric really helped give my skin a vibrant glow. I was thrilled to discover other natural plants that can truly clean the blood and enhance the skin. I loved the spirit of the people of India, and to this day it remains one of my favorite countries.

When I finally made my way to Africa, I was mesmerized by the gorgeous, velvety skin of African women. From teenagers to women well into their sixties, they had poreless and perfectly moisturized complexions, without a zit or wrinkle in sight. I discovered that in countries like Ethiopia they use raw shea butter on their skin, which comes from a native nut and is scraped out fresh. It furthered my belief that pure and natural moisturizers are far superior to synthetic, petroleum-based ones, which most women in the Western world use. Diet issues aside, I realized that with our plethora of eye creams, serums, sunscreens and thick, heavy night creams, American women are *suffocating* their skin. I decided right then that I would take the cue from African women and use natural skin products that truly nourish the skin and allow it to breathe.

When I came back from my world journey, it was not easy for me to integrate back into American life. I was trying to put it all together and figure out how to combine my passion for skin care, health and nutrition. The first thing I did was get a job at one of the biggest beauty companies in the world. I wanted an inside glimpse into the beauty world to see if I could use my experiences there. But big corporate beauty was definitely not for me. I did, however, get a great education about the industry, and I learned some tricks of the trade that provided me with a foundation from which to make my dream of running my own company a reality.

I pursued my insatiable thirst for natural health and beauty information to further the teachings I learned abroad. I decided to start a small beauty company, which took a few years to get up and running—and a whole lot of patience and work! During this time, I worked at various jobs to support myself, including as a yoga instructor (I still teach, because I love it so much!) and a brief stint as a model. I became a certified clinical nutritionist and worked at a longevity center in Manhattan to further my knowledge of nutrition and natural healing. I also studied at various natural health institutions, including the Ann Wigmore Natural Health Institute in Puerto Rico.

With my first venture, I learned the ropes of running my own business. It was a great learning experience. But soon I was pulled in the direction of a much larger mission in life:

to share my passion for health and beauty with others in a much broader way. I started a health and beauty blog (www.kimberlysnyder.net), which grew quickly by word of mouth and soon started attracting a lot of press and media attention. I began conducting private nutritional counseling sessions and working with A-list celebrities (and on location at some of Hollywood's biggest film sets), counseling them on how to improve and balance their diets through cleansing. Throughout the book I share stories of some of my actual clients so that you can see the sorts of incredible results this program achieves. Of course, their real names have been changed for privacy.

It was clear from the response to my blog and nutritional counseling that there is an enormous hunger out there for the information I was sharing, and it became clear to me that I needed to do something to help people on a larger scale. It was this hunger that was the true inspiration for this book. It also became evident to me that as part of this mission I needed to create a forum devoted to sharing information and ideas encompassing *all* aspects of health, beauty, nutrition, and wellness. The inspiration to create a Beauty Detox community was born, and I expanded my blog into a website, where people can interact, ask questions and support each other. In the future, I am also inspired to create some products that I can 100% get behind that will also help people achieve their highest level of beauty and health, including skincare, probiotics and digestive enzymes. Because I am so incredibly selective about the quality of ingredients and formulations, it might take a little time, but it will happen!

The Beauty Detox Solution and the Beauty Detox Community reflect the heart and soul of the lessons I learned during my world journey and studies, and my passion for health. As I learned from the beautiful women of Africa, I don't advocate slathering tons of products on your skin or following complicated skin-care programs just because I want to make some extra bucks pushing unnecessary products. I want our largest organ, the skin, to breathe, and I also want women to look to the internal root causes of beauty issues to fix them, rather than mask these problems with makeup or prescription drugs. We can eat and cleanse our way to profound beauty. The right products can greatly support this, but the right diet is critical to the overall program.

From my three-year world journey and subsequent years of study, I discovered the truth about health and beauty: the healthiest tools, those that will enable us all to achieve our most beautiful selves, are born in nature and are right there for the taking. The answer is so simple: it is about eating the right foods in the right way to ensure we are consistently cleansing our bodies of toxins and getting all the beauty nutrients we need to look our best.

We don't have to starve or deprive ourselves, and we can eat abundantly. By keeping to the simple principles that I outline for you in this book, you will reach new levels of beauty and energy that will amaze you. You can look better in your thirties, forties and fifties than you did in your twenties and thirties, and *feel* better.

In Part 1 of this book I outline the broad concepts of detoxing for beauty, and in Part 2 I outline the actual phases, meal plans and recipes for you to create your own beauty solution. I recognize that we're all at different levels of health. For this reason, I've created three Beauty Detox phases: Blossoming Beauty, Radiant Beauty and True Beauty. There is one phase to fit everyone. I did *not* design the Beauty Detox Solution to be a three-step program. If you feel great as a Blossoming Beauty, then you might want to stay there. Or perhaps you're inspired to move into True Beauty. This is not a race or a competition—start with the phase that's right for you and progress at your own pace. This is not a short-term diet, but rather a lifestyle program.

Whenever I start working with a new client, before I make any dietary changes what-soever, I always begin by explaining the concepts in Part 1. Understanding the concepts in Part 1 is critical to making this program work for you, especially since a lot of the concepts may be new to you. Reading all the information in Part 1 is essential to following the Beauty Detox and will ensure you see the results you want.

The information in this book is different from that in any other diet or detox book you may read. It is a hybrid of knowledge I've acquired from many different teachers, health institutions and training programs, as well as from my around-the-world journey.

Some of the principles we will discuss have not yet trickled into mainstream health and nutrition practices, but the concepts presented here are based on the sound, thorough research and work of many doctors, scientists and research institutions. I have cited numer-ous studies and specific research throughout for your reference, so that you can see how the science supports the program.

Keep an open mind as you read, and remember that many tenets of health that are widely accepted now—like how smoking cigarettes increases your odds of getting lung cancer—

were not always mainstream ideas. Set aside the myriad of confusing and conflicting health concepts that you have internalized from various media, health magazines, doctors and family members. If you keep an open mind and listen to your intuition, you can discover the true secrets to beauty.

Reading this book will open up a whole new way for you to understand the powerful connection between food, health and beauty. *The Beauty Detox Solution* will take you to your most beautiful, energetic, healthy self. When I started my personal Beauty Detox, it changed my life—and I know this book can do the same for you. I'm so excited for you!

With Love and Best Wishes for True Beauty,
Kimberly

THE
BEAUTY
DETOX
SOLUTION

PART ONE

BEAUTY **DETOX** BASICS

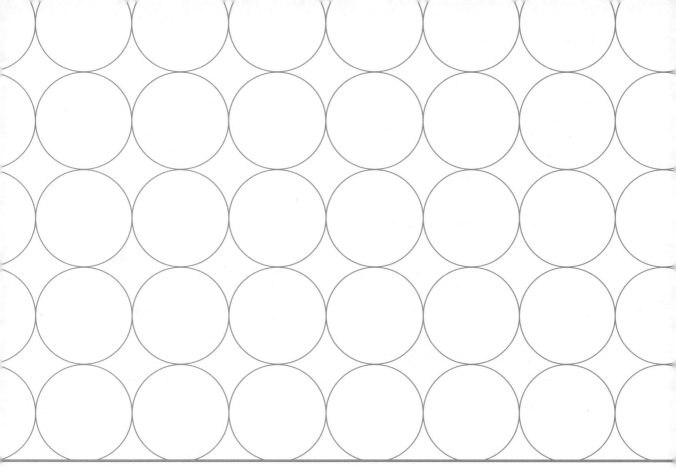

CHAPTER ONE

OUR DIET, DICTATED BY NATURE

In order to Become Younger, many of one's habits must be changed. To do this constructively, one can do it only with an open mind and with the wholehearted desire to see if it really works.

A closed mind...a mind which has made it a practice to frown on radical changes in thought, habits and actions, is the greatest stumbling block towards any progress on the road to Become Younger.

— Dr. Norman Walker
Become Younger

The connection between food and beauty is incredibly powerful—just by changing the foods you eat, you can radically change the way you look and feel. So our discussion begins with a very basic question: what are we designed to eat? And to answer it, we have to know where we as humans belong in nature. Not in a philosophical, "new age" sense, but in a physical, anatomical sense. We can't do calculus until we know how to add nine and three, and so it is in all aspects of life. Let's first take a step back and examine our place within the animal kingdom and nature.

HOW OUR BODY IS DESIGNED

One of the best ways to figure out where we belong is to look at the animal kingdom. The human body is most closely related to that of primates: monkeys, chimps (like Tarzan's sidekick) and gorillas. Our genetic makeup is more similar to that of chimpanzees than to that of any other species on the planet, with an estimated 99.4 percent of our DNA sequence shared.[1]

Look down at your hands, which are holding this book. Don't they look similar to monkeys' hands? Look at your nails, flexible fingers and opposable thumbs. Now grind your teeth back and forth. You'll find that our teeth, like monkeys', are flattened (except the front canines, which can be used to help open up the harder shells of some fruits). Our back molars are appropriate for grinding plants for easy digestion.

Carnivorous animals, like the tiger, for example, have short, inflexible "fingers," which are really protrusions to push out and retract claws. These claws are needed to rip into the flesh of their prey. The tiger and other carnivores have sharp fangs: even their back molars are sharp and pointed, perfect for hunting and eating raw meat. *Without* these claws and sharp teeth, it would be impossible for the tiger to feast on its prey. Our hands, teeth and bodies simply aren't designed for hunting and devouring animals in the same way; we have to use tools, weapons and utensils instead.

Okay, so we *look* different. But it turns out that our digestive tract is built differently, as well. The human liver, for instance, has a low tolerance for uric acid, a by-product of digesting animal protein. In contrast, the liver of the carnivorous tiger contains uricase, which is an enzyme used to break down uric acid. This enzyme gives the carnivorous tiger's liver about fifteen times the capacity to break down uric acid from animal protein than a human liver has.

Not only are our livers designed to digest plant foods, but our stomachs are, too. The stomach juices of the tiger and other carnivores have a very high concentration of acid. This high concentration of acid helps to quickly and efficiently break down the high concentration of proteins that make up the carnivore's diet. Humans' stomach acid, on the other hand, is much less concentrated. Carnivores' stomach acid is at least ten times more concentrated, and some researchers believe it could be many times more concentrated than that.

And what is true in the liver and stomach is true in the rest of the digestive tract. The human intestine is extremely complex, and at around thirty feet, it is about twelve times as long as our torso. (The gorilla also has a long intestine—about eight to twelve times its torso length.) It is designed to be long so there is adequate time to absorb the minerals and nutrients of fruits and plant matter, which quickly break down and move through our bodies much faster than animal protein does. The carnivorous tiger, on the other hand, has a short intestine—only about three times the length of its torso. Its intestinal tract is designed for quickly getting rid of the acidic waste matter that is the by-product of animal protein.

HOW OUR DESIGN AFFECTS OUR DIET

Now we've taken a quick look at where we belong in the animal kingdom. So what does this mean for our diet?

The gorilla is a natural vegetarian, and 86 percent of its diet is composed of green leaves, shoots and stems, with the other 14 percent made up primarily of bark, roots, flowers and fruit.[2] The gorilla gets all its protein, vitamin and mineral needs from its plant-based diet and is in fact the strongest animal on earth, pound for pound.

In contrast, the tiger is a full-blooded carnivore and lives off other animals' flesh to derive its nutrition. Its organs are efficiently designed for quickly breaking down and expelling heavy fat and protein molecules, as well as the by-products of their digestion. A tiger's speedy digestive system keeps the tiger from becoming toxic and sick from its very acidic diet. Its body uses what it needs and gets the rest of the garbage out…fast!

So what happens when we have the biological makeup of a gorilla but we eat like a tiger? Trouble! We are going against the natural laws of biology.

What does this mean for your health and beauty? The key to being your healthiest, more beautiful self is eating the way your body was designed to eat. As you'll discover in more detail in Chapter 4, fruits and vegetables have powerful minerals and enzymes that promote beauty from the inside out. And it's well documented that loading up on plant foods and cutting back on animal protein help us slim down. At the Pritikin Longevity Center in Florida, forty-five hundred patients who went through a three-week program and were given a mostly plant-based diet and who exercised lost 5.5 percent of their body weight.[3]

Where We Belong in Nature

	Humans	Gorillas	Tigers
Hands	Nimble fingers, with flattened nails perfect for pulling down and eating fruits	Nimble fingers, with flattened nails perfect for pulling down and eating fruits	Short, inflexible fingers with sharp claws that tear into and rip apart animal prey
Teeth	Flattened for grinding plant matter, especially back molars	Front teeth sharp for opening up fruit shells and tearing down plants, back teeth flattened for grinding plant matter	Long, sharp and pointed fangs, with sharp back molars
Liver	Low tolerance for uric acid, which is a by-product of digesting animal protein	Low tolerance for uric acid, which is a by-product of digesting animal protein	Contains uricase, to break down uric acid, which is a by-product of digesting animal protein
Intestines	At least twelve times as long as trunk, which provides a long transit time to extract minerals and nutrients from plant foods	About eight to twelve times as long as trunk, which provides a long transit time to extract minerals and nutrients from plant foods	Only three times as long as trunk, designed to rapidly expel waste matter
Stomach	Low concentration of acid, perfect for breaking down plant matter	Low concentration of acid, perfect for breaking down plant matter	High concentration of acid to break down animal protein

Eating too much animal protein actually strips your body of beauty, because digestion of protein produces toxins in the body. This makes sense when you think about how your body works. It causes a great strain on your liver to process all the uric acid created from digesting animal protein. And that's big trouble, because your liver has a lot of work to do: your liver is the largest internal organ, and it's in charge of metabolizing fat and cleansing the body of toxins.

Your long intestinal tract is simply not designed to process large amounts of meat. When you put large amounts of heavy animal protein in your long intestine, the protein just hobbles along as best it can, which isn't very fast, since it has to pass through the winding corridors of so many feet of intestine. Because it takes so long in that hot environment, it can start to putrefy, or, in other words, rot, causing unhealthy bacterial growth and toxicity. There is no other way to put it: waste from digested animal products is meant to exit the body quickly, as it does in a carnivore's body, not linger in your long digestive tract.

Digesting protein creates all sorts of by-products in the body, like purines, uric acid and ammonia, all of which create acidity in the body. These toxins are absorbed into our bloodstream through the colon and circulate all around our bodies. When our blood is clogged with toxins, it can't transport as many beautifying minerals, and these toxins can age and clog the skin cells of our face. In his book *Conscious Eating,* Gabriel Cousens, M.D., discusses how ammonia, a by-product of digesting protein, contributes to aging. As he states, "Ammonia, which is a breakdown product of a high-flesh-food diet, is directly toxic to the system. It has been found to create free radical damage and cross-linking (a process associated with skin wrinkles and aging), as well as depletes the body's energy."[4]

Our bodies are cleverly designed for survival, and one of the most important ways to do that is to protect the vital organs. As renowned microbiologist Dr. Robert Young points out, one way the body does

The Strongest Animals on Earth Are Vegetarian

The gorilla—a vegetarian by nature and design—is the strongest animal on earth, pound for pound. The same is true of other large and strong mammals on earth—the elephant, hippopotamus, giraffe, rhinoceros, wild horse, buffalo. *They are all plant eaters.* Imagine that! All these really strong, gigantic animals get *all* their protein needs from the amino acids, the building blocks of protein, in plants. That is solid proof in nature that vegetarians can not only get more than enough protein but can also build large, defined muscles.

Evolving Choices, Evolving Beauty

You might be wondering why, if eating plant foods is so natural for humans, we have been eating meat for thousands of years. Yes, humans have been eating meat for many generations, very often for survival, but that doesn't mean that it's ideal for us to eat. Our ancestors had to survive off anything they could pick or catch. Life spans and living conditions were completely different many generations ago. And our ancestors supplemented their diets with numerous plant foods—and they certainly didn't eat meat in the amounts traditionally eaten in the Western world today!

When we know better, we do better. Not only do we have more knowledge today, but we have more choices. We have access to grocery stores, food co-ops and farmers' markets and can choose from a wide variety of foods. With these wide choices that are available to us, we don't have to worry about merely surviving anymore. We have the amazing opportunity to reach our ultimate beauty potential and live a life that is long and disease free.

this is by expanding fat cells to store acidic and toxic waste, to keep it away from our organs.[5] This is one reason detoxing will help you lose weight. The body won't let go of excess fat that's protecting you from your own toxins! But as you begin to cleanse yourself of toxic, acidic waste, as well as fat-soluble chemicals found in many processed foods,[6] you can shed the pesky extra pounds much easier. The more toxicity you have in your body, the faster you age and the more you will struggle with maintaining your ideal weight.

Let's return for a moment to the question we opened with: where do human beings fit in nature? We now have an answer. We are designed to eat a diet primarily made up of plant foods: greens, fruits and vegetables, sprouts, seeds and nuts. With this type of diet, we flourish and derive all our necessary nutrients, while also keeping our bodies toxin free and looking our most beautiful. This is the basis of the Beauty Detox Solution—you will be filling your body with nourishing plant foods that are chock-full of Beauty Minerals and other key nutrients that will make you more beautiful from the inside out.

If we want to reach our highest goals and achieve True Beauty, we have to work with nature. Many of us load up on animal protein, probably because we've been taught that we need animal protein to "be healthy," and that we must "get enough protein" to feed our muscles and tissues. Just think about it. If we were designed to eat so much animal protein, why are so many people getting fatter and fatter, and sicker and sicker, and visibly aging so fast that Botox injections and face-lifts are now commonplace procedures? It is because we are going against nature's inherent laws. Aging at the fast rate most people age is *not* inevitable.

Don't worry. You will be getting more than enough protein on the Beauty Detox Solution, but it will be derived from beautifying plant foods.

THE SCIENCE BEHIND THE BEAUTY DETOX SOLUTION

What I've told you so far has been mainly observational, but there's also significant scientific evidence supporting the benefits of a plant-based, low-acid diet. And there's more and more research coming out on how dangerous a diet high in animal protein really is.

There are over thirty-five hundred scientific studies involving over fifteen thousand research scientists that report a relationship between the consumption of meats, poultry, eggs and dairy products and the incidence of numerous health issues, including but not restricted to heart disease, cancer, kidney failure, constipation, gout, gallstones, diverticulosis, hemorrhoids and osteoporosis. This research could fill this whole book alone! Here I'll list a few landmark studies and the work of researchers that I think are so important that everyone should know about their findings.

A Note for Meat Lovers

If you love to eat meat, don't panic! *You do not have to become a full-fledged vegetarian if you don't want to.* Throughout this book I share research into the nutritional benefits of eating a more vegetarian diet and explain how a vegetarian diet is ideal for cleansing, but I know that many people won't want to give up meat entirely. And that's okay. You can still reap the incredible benefits of the Beauty Detox Solution while incorporating meat and other animal products into your diet. Throughout the book I'll help you determine the best kinds of meat to eat and the best way to eat meat to support your Beauty Detox.

CANCER RISK

A major review on diet and cancer prepared for the U.S. Congress in 1981 estimated that genetics determines only about 2 to 3 percent of the total cancer risk.[12] That's why the incredible findings of the China-Cornell-Oxford Project, simply known as the China Project, are important to note. The China Project was the most comprehensive study on the connection between diet and disease in medical history. Funded by such prestigious organizations as the National Institutes of Health, the American Cancer Society and the American Institute for Cancer Research, and spearheaded by T. Colin Campbell, Ph.D., a professor in the Division of Nutritional Sciences at Cornell University and a former senior science advisor to the American Institute for Cancer Research, the China Project was launched in the early 1980s and ran for nearly thirty years. Dr. Camp-

How Much Protein Do We Really Need?

The World Health Organization recommends that only about 5 percent of our daily calories be from protein.[7] Incidentally, that is the same percentage of protein as in human breast milk.

The RDA recommendation from the Institute of Medicine is that we take in about 0.8 grams of protein per kilogram that we weigh.[8] This recommendation includes a generous safety factor for most people.

The prominent nutrition expert Dr. John Scharffenberg gave an extensive presentation at the annual meeting of the American Association for the Advancement of Science, which was ultimately published in 1982. He was quoted as saying, "Let me emphasize, it is difficult to design a reasonable experimental diet that provides an active adult with adequate calories that is deficient in protein."[9] Nathan Pritikin, the founder of the Pritikin Longevity Center in Florida, whose work has proven the incredible healing powers of a plant-based diet, once stated, "Vegetarians always ask about getting enough protein. But I don't know any nutrition expert that can plan a diet of natural foods resulting in a protein deficiency, so long as you're not deficient in calories. You need only six percent of total calories in protein...and it's practically impossible to get below nine percent in ordinary diets."[10]

While there may be many different opinions on the exact amount of protein we need, one thing is clear: the average plant food supplies at least 10 percent of its calories in the form of protein, and green vegetables average about 50 percent.[11] You can rest assured that on the Beauty Detox Solution, which is whole-food based and plant based, with a ton of greens, you will be getting plenty of protein! I go into more detail on this in Chapter 5.

bell's research found more than eight thousand statistically significant associations between various dietary factors and disease. Dr. Campbell's findings were ultimately published in his book *The China Study*.

Most notably, the China Project revealed a strong correlation between cancer and animal protein and dairy consumption.[13] As Dr. Campbell explains in *The China Study*, "dietary protein proved to be so powerful in its effect that we could turn on and turn off cancer growth simply by changing the level consumed." The China Project, along with some seven hundred and fifty studies Campbell cites in *The China Study*, demonstrably revealed that a plant-based diet supplies more than adequate protein and calcium, as well as other important minerals and nutrients needed for health. It also pinpointed the powerful connection between diet—namely, eating animal-based foods—and disease. As Dr. Campbell summarizes: "Plant-based foods are linked to lower blood cholesterol; animal-based foods are linked to higher blood cholesterol. Animal-based foods are linked to higher breast cancer rates; plant-based foods are linked to lower rates. Fiber and antioxidants from plants are linked to a lower risk of cancers of the digestive tract. Plant-based diets and active lifestyles result in a healthy weight, yet permit people to become big and strong."[14]

HEART DISEASE

Heart disease is currently the number one cause of death for both men and women in America. According to the American Heart Association,[20] cardiovascular disease affects over eighty-one million Americans for a stunning total of 37 percent of the American population.[21]

Dr. Dean Ornish is a Harvard Medical School graduate and a pioneer in the connection between heart disease and diet. Dr. Ornish headed up the research in the Lifestyle Heart Trial,[22] in which he treated twenty-eight heart disease patients with lifestyle changes alone, without any medications or surgery. For a year the twenty-eight patients in the experimental group were asked to eat a plant-based, low-fat diet (about 10 percent of their daily calories coming from fat). They could eat as much food as they wanted from the allowable food list, which contained primarily greens and other vegetables, whole grains and fruit. No animal food products were allowed at all, except some egg white and a maximum of one cup of nonfat milk or yogurt per day. The patients exercised three hours a week and practiced various forms of stress management, like meditation and breathing exercises. During this year Dr. Ornish also tracked a control group of twenty patients that were put on a standard treatment plan for heart disease.

The results were nothing short of fantastic. Eighty-two percent of the patients in the experimental group that were eating the plant-based diet had a regression in their heart disease over the course of the year. The blockages in their arteries diminished. This group had a 91 percent reduction in the frequency of chest pain, their total cholesterol dropped on average from 227 mg/dL to 172 mg/dL and, on average, their "bad" LDL cholesterol fell from 152 mg/dL to 95 mg/dL. In contrast, those in the control group, who received the standard care, saw a 165 percent rise in the frequency of chest pain. Their cholesterol levels were significantly worse than those of members of the experimental group, and the blockages in their arteries increased by up to 8 percent.

This success inspired Dr. Ornish to expand the Lifestyle Heart Trial into the Multi-center Lifestyle Demonstration Project.[23] Patients with serious heart disease enrolled in a one-year lifestyle program as an alternative to heart surgery. By 1998 two hundred people had taken part in the program. After one year of treatment chest pain was eliminated for 65 percent of patients, and after three years 60 percent of the patients continued reporting no chest pain. We can see from Dr. Ornish's research how a plant-based diet with little to no animal products has serious implications for the battle against heart disease and the restoration of health.

DIABETES

Another disease we should touch upon is diabetes. According to the American Diabetes Association, as of 2007 over 23.6 million Americans have diabetes, which is roughly 8 percent of the American population.[24] Type 2 diabetes (also known as adult-onset diabetes, though it's becoming more and more prevalent in younger individuals) is on the rise. Diabetes treatments cost something to the tune of $174 billion in the United States in 2007.[25] Besides greatly increasing the risk for heart disease, stroke and high blood pressure, type 2 diabetes comes with such terrifying complications as blindness, amputation and kidney disease.

The good news is that studies show that the diet we choose to eat can not only prevent diabetes, but it can treat diabetes, as well. Dr. James Anderson is a prominent medical doctor studying diabetes and its treatment with diet. One study he conducted examined the effects of a mostly plant-food diet that was rich in fiber and carbohydrates and low in fat.[26] It involved twenty-five type 1 diabetics and twenty-five type 2 diabetics in a controlled hospital setting. (Type 1 diabetics cannot produce insulin, and it would seem far less likely that these patients would garner any benefit from a dietary change alone.) All the participants were not overweight, and 100 percent of them were taking insulin shots to regulate their blood sugar levels. For the first week all the patients were fed the standard diet recommended by the American Diabetes Association, which included meat and dairy products. For the next three weeks the patients switched over to a plant-based, mostly vegetarian diet. Dr. Anderson then studied the effect of the new diet on the patients' blood sugar and cholesterol levels, as well as on their weight and medication requirements.

Plant Foods Decrease Colon Cancer Risk

According to the International Agency for Research on Cancer (IARC), which is part of the World Health Organization, colorectal cancer is the third most common cancer in men and the second most common cancer in women worldwide. Almost 60 percent of the cases occur in developed regions.[15] In one study researchers compared environmental factors and cancer rates in thirty-two countries and found a strong correlation between colon cancer and meat intake.[16] This study found in particular that regions where more animal protein, more sugar and fewer cereal grains were consumed had far higher rates of colon cancer.[17]

Studies show that eating more fiber—which is found in plant foods *only*—decreases your risk of colon cancer. A large study in 2003 by the European Prospective Investigation into Cancer and Nutrition (EPIC)[18] collected data on fiber intake and colorectal cancer in five hundred nineteen thousand people across Europe and found that the 20 percent of people that consumed the most fiber in their diet (about thirty-four grams per day), had a 42 percent lower risk of colorectal cancer than the 20 percent who consumed the least fiber in their diet (about thirteen grams a day).[19]

Given its widespread prevalence, colon cancer affects all of us. I have many fond memories spending time as a child with my grandmother on my father's side, Nana, who taught me how to knit and paint with acrylic and oil paints on canvas. Nana took her fiber supplement every day but did not eat a lot of vegetables and fruits that are naturally high in fiber. Nana passed away from colon cancer in 1996, at the young age of sixty-four.

True Beauty Story

BARBARA MULREADY IS A CLIENT OF MINE IN HER EARLY FORTIES. SHE IS TALL, with long blond hair, has a fit body and stays within five pounds of her ideal weight. However, when I met her, she had very shallow, dark circles under her eyes, which gave her a permanently tired expression. The nasolabial fold between her nose and her mouth was also very deep, and her cheeks looked sunken. The words that come to mind to describe how she looked at that first meeting we had at a tea café were unfortunately "beat down."

Ironically, Barbara is a personal trainer. She gives advice to *her* clients on how to eat, but she could tell something was off with her own diet, and she sought out my help. Her energy was very low, she was often irritable and emotional, and she did not have regular, adequate bowel movements. When I looked into her eyes, I saw a deflated version of the real Barbara, as if a wet cloth had been laid over her true radiance.

When I looked at her diet, I saw that she was eating small meals five to seven times a day, and that most of her mini meals included some kind of lean animal protein. As a result of eating such a high-protein, acidic diet, outwardly her body was fairly toned and thin, but inwardly she was aging at an accelerated rate, as told by her shallow, uneven skin and constant struggle to get through the day.

As a personal trainer and gym rat, she was led to believe that she had to constantly consume animal protein—chicken breast, egg white, tuna, whey protein, etc.—in order to maintain her muscle tone and get the most out of her workouts. But she never learned how acidic this type of diet made her body. We started transitioning her diet to incorporate more easily assimilated sources of plant protein, such as hemp protein and high-protein algae (chlorella) tablets, after her workouts and started cutting back on the amount of acidic animal products she consumed. We started with small steps, and she quickly saw her energy increase and her skin improve.

Today Barbara still eats some animal protein—she loves fish, eggs and some chicken—but she eats nowhere *near* the amount of these foods that she used to eat. She also shifted to eating those foods later on in the day. Ironically, her body became even more toned as old acidic waste was eliminated and oxygen was able to circulate to her muscles more as there was now less pressure on her veins and arteries from gas created by fermentation. Her energy is now so high that she lasts all the way into the night without any caffeine, and her skin has drastically improved, achieving a healthy glow. Her blond hair now has a healthy sheen, as opposed to the brittleness it once had, and the circles under her eyes have greatly reduced. She looks years younger. And yes, she is now going to the bathroom regularly! Best of all, she is smiling and laughing again, and she feels much younger, lighter and happier.

After just three weeks on the plant-based diet, the type 1 diabetic patients were able to lower their insulin medication by an average of 40 percent. Blood sugar profiles greatly improved, and their cholesterol levels dropped by 30 percent.[27] Of the twenty-five patients with type 2 diabetes, twenty-four were able to discontinue their insulin medication![28] That means only *one* out of twenty-five type 2 diabetics in the study had to stay on insulin medication as a result of switching to a plant-based, high-fiber and low-fat diet for only three weeks!

A group of research scientists at the Pritikin Center also studied the effects of a plant-based diet low in fat, along with exercise, on diabetic patients. Of the forty patients that were all on medication at the start of the program, thirty-four were able to discontinue all medication after only twenty-six days.[29]

The Grand World War Experiments

Not all studies into the benefits of a plant-based diet take place in a lab. Some come directly from history.

During World War I, Denmark was cut off from all imports, including food, by the allied blockade. Dr. Mikkel Hindhede was appointed by the Danish government to develop a program for the country to avoid the crisis of a major food shortage. Dr. Hindhede stopped feeding the country's grain to livestock and instead fed it directly to the people to conserve the food supply. It was pretty much a national experiment in vegetarianism, involving the three million citizens of Denmark. Dr. Hindhede later reported his findings in the *Journal of the American Medical Association* (*JAMA*).[30]

The results were incredible. During the period when the food restrictions were the most severe, which was from October 1917 to October 1918, the death rate in Copenhagen from disease was by far the lowest in recorded history. In fact, it decreased over 34 percent when compared to figures for the preceding eighteen years![31]

During World War II Norway was occupied by Germany, and Norway had to sharply reduce and often eliminate the meat distribution to its people. Once again, amazing improvements in health occurred.[32] The death rate from circulatory disease dropped dramatically. When the war ended and the Norwegian citizens went back to their normal diet, which included meat, the death rate rose again[33] almost with perfect mathematical precision.

Britain also had a significant decrease in its consumption of meat and other animal products during World War II. Reports were in keeping with the massive health improvements found in Denmark and Norway during their near-vegetarian periods. There were many signs of general improved health, including a drop in the prevalence of anemia and a significant decrease in infant and postnatal deaths.[34]

All are compelling examples of how much health can improve with a vegetarian diet.

The findings of these studies are unquestionably impressive and support the theory that a plant-based diet will bolster our beauty and health. And more and more medical doctors are becoming aware of the overwhelming long-term scientific data that prove that our bodies can and will flourish on plant food. Prominent doctors who promote a plant-based diet include Dr. John McDougall, Dr. Kerrie Saunders, Dr. Caldwell Esselstyn and Dr. Joel Fuhrman, who is on the board of the National Health Association. The Physicians Committee for Responsible Medicine, which boasts a membership of over five thousand physicians, was founded by Dr. Neal Barnard and has prominent medical doctors, such as Dr. Andrew Weil, on its advisory board. It has reexamined nutritional criteria and strongly advocates a vegan diet, which it believes helps combat a multitude of physical health ailments, including heart disease, cancer, stroke and diabetes.[35] It is leading the way for improved federal nutritional policies.

Again, you don't have to become a vegetarian or vegan for the Beauty Detox Solution to work for you. Even if you still eat animal protein, your intake of plant food will dramatically increase. And you can rest assured that by shifting into a more plant-based diet, your body will become an efficiently operating machine, and you will amass far less internal toxicity. You will become more beautiful and vibrant!

Now that we have begun our discussion with a firm understanding of our place in nature and the incredible benefits of eating plant-based foods, you're ready to discover the secrets to radiant health and beauty.

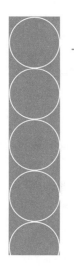

BEAUTY **DETOX** RECAP

- ○ Humans resemble herbivores, in terms of both their anatomical structure and internal organs.
- ○ Our intestines and digestive tract are designed to reap the full benefits of amino acids, minerals and other nutrients from plant foods.
- ○ We will slow down aging and look younger if we limit our intake of animal protein and increase our intake of plant foods.
- ○ Studies show that there is a strong correlation between eating animal protein and the incidence of cancer, heart disease and other illnesses.

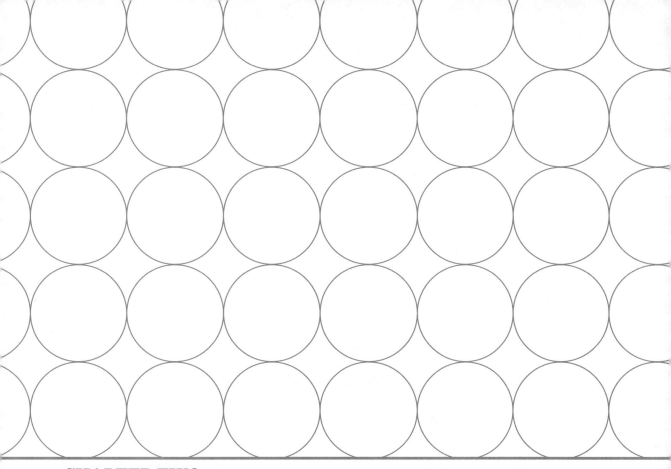

CHAPTER TWO

BEAUTY ENERGY

Medicines have limitations; the divine creative life force has none.

—Swami Sri Yukteswar

One of the most important assets we have in our quest for beauty is energy. Energy is a key factor in our ability to shed weight easily and permanently, achieve great health and look our most beautiful. Let's refer to all the energy the body spends to do these amazing things as "Beauty Energy." Where do we get our energy? From food, clean air, sunlight and, depending on your spiritual beliefs, a higher power.

Our energy is more precious than all the gold in the world. It is a more powerful anti-aging tool than face-lifts, Botox, Restylane, or anything else. Energy fuels how efficiently our organs work, how efficiently we detox our bodies, and how efficiently our body is able to do the very basic things that contribute to beauty. Energy regenerates our liver and other tissue cells, flushes toxic waste from the body, helps maintain our ideal weight, keeps our skin's collagen smooth and our hair healthy, and keeps blood from stagnating into dark under-eye circles! The more energy we have, the better we feel and the more beautiful we become.

MORE ENERGY = MORE BEAUTY

What eats up energy? Most of us first think of physical activities when we consider what exhausts our energy: walking, running and going to the gym. But beyond that, the amazing machine of the human body organizes our billions of cells as it performs an astonishing number of internal functions on a constant daily basis.

Let's focus on one of those functions: *digestion*. Yes, digestion! Did you know that the full process of digestion takes more energy than any other specific internal function of the human body? Some experts estimate that digestion takes as much as 50 to 80 percent of our total energy.[1]

Imagine that your body keeps all its energy in a pantry, just as you keep your food in one. Picture containers of various sizes holding energy dedicated to the body's different activities—rebuilding collagen in the skin, cleansing, growing hair and nails. In the middle of the pantry is a container that is far, far bigger than all the others—and big enough to hold more than half of the total energy in the pantry. That is the energy the body uses for digestion.

Digestion is the key that can elevate our beauty to the highest levels, or, adversely, take us down, by sucking up precious energy that could be used for other processes. The Beauty Detox Solution is designed to free up energy from digestion, which is the single most important way to redirect large amounts of energy to make weight loss easy and help us look our most beautiful.

THE REAL CAUSE OF AGING

Most people try to fight aging by getting fillers or face-lifts, avoiding so much as a drop of sunlight on their faces without some kind of sunscreen, using increasingly more expensive antiwrinkle creams, eating fatty fish or other animal proteins to "plump or support the skin"... or finally giving up the fight altogether. The problem is not that aging is inevitable; it is that most of us don't understand what really *causes* aging.

The analogy I always like to use is to think of ourselves as wheels. When we are children, the wheel rolls along quickly and easily, and without obstruction. We never had to obsess over what to eat, or how many calories or grams of carbs we were ingesting, yet we were always the right weight, had high energy, and slept perfectly. Over time, from years of exposure to less than perfect foods, pollution, preservatives, toxic additives, medications and many other things, waste begins to build up in our bodies.

Internal waste is like sludge in the spokes of a wheel. Think of dirt or mud that gets kicked up into the spokes of a wheel and then hardens and sticks over time to create sludge. The sludge stuck in the spokes of the wheel prevents the wheel from rolling along powerfully and easily. The wheel slows down. As the years go by, it becomes increasingly harder to maintain your weight or have high energy— even if you were eating the same exact way five years earlier. Suddenly issues begin to

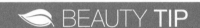

BEAUTY TIP

Grow Younger

If I met you six weeks ago and said hello, and we met again today, most or all the cells on your face would be brand-new. That's because every six to eight weeks the skin cells on our face are renewed. In fact, *most* of the cells of our body are replaced each year. Bone and dentin can be around seven years old, but most of the body's cells are much newer than that.[2] That's great news for us, because even if we have lived a life of abuse and poor habits, much of that is reversible if we begin to adopt good habits and consistently build on them *now*.

Following the Beauty Detox Solution will give your body the best quality nutrition while simultaneously cleansing your cells on an ongoing basis. Minerals and nutrients will be absorbed by your body more efficiently, your cells will become more purified and you will look younger. Puffiness, chronic dark under-eye circles and wrinkles will start to melt away.

Forget the past, what you've heard, and what your chronological age is. It is possible to grow younger, not older! And it *is* possible to look and feel better now than you did one or even a few decades ago.

pop up in many different forms, ranging from the inconvenient ones, like acne or brittle nails, to the life-threatening ones, like various diseases.

This sludge is what makes us old. We can throw expensive supplements, prescription antiaging creams, or Botox on top of it all day long, but we will never fully be able to fight aging unless and until we work to *clean out the sludge.*

This sludge is what slows our body down, and it is also a primary factor in the speed at which we age and in our ability to keep excess weight off. I know people that eat the Beauty Detox Solution way that are fifty-three and look thirty-five. One woman I know is thirty-seven and looks as if she can't possibly be older than her midtwenties. It *is* possible.

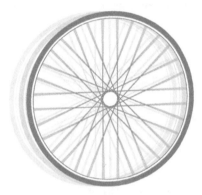

**Healthy and Youthful:
The wheel rolls along easily,
with no obstruction.**

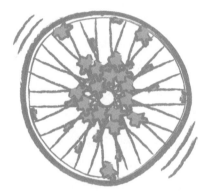

**The Cause of Aging: Cemented,
hardened sludge in the spokes of
the wheel, which makes the wheel
and all its functions slow down.**

A CLEAN BODY IS A BEAUTIFUL BODY

I speak of beauty and health interchangeably, and it is a natural law that you cannot be truly and fully beautiful until you are in superior health. The great natural healing pioneer Professor Arnold Ehret wrote, "Disease is an effort of the body to eliminate waste, mucus and toxemias, and this system assists Nature in the most perfect and natural way. Not the disease but the body is to be healed; it must be cleansed, freed from waste and foreign matter, from mucus and toxemias accumulated since childhood."[3]

Our body's systems are always trying to maintain perfect balance, which leads to the most superb health and beauty, but this is only truly possible once we have cleansed ourselves of toxic material—both the old sludge and the new sludge that accumulates constantly. Why? It all comes down to digestion and how much Beauty Energy we have.

Remember that our bodies are designed for survival, so the energy will go first to maintain our life-sustaining processes and internal organs. Keeping our skin wrinkle free and our hair shiny is of little concern to our bodies when our livers are overloaded with waste, our adrenals are exhausted and our intestines are all backed up!

Now that you know how much energy the body spends to digest food, it makes sense that the more efficiently we digest food (or the less energy the body has to spend on digesting), the *more* energy the body has to clean out the old toxic material and perform all those beautifying process. The toxic sludge amasses at a much faster pace when we are not digesting our food efficiently.

Detoxing ourselves by getting rid of old waste is key to allowing our digestion to function optimally. When we loosen the toxic sludge from the spokes of the wheel, our energy will

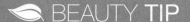

BEAUTY TIP

Eat Your Way to a Wrinkle-Free Face

Traditional Chinese medicine tells us that our face is a window into the vitality of organs in the body, and that there are meridians, or energy pathways, running all throughout the body. In a similar vein, in the Western tradition we learn that there are reflexes, or nerve pathways, that run throughout the body. Reflexes trigger an impulse to go through the point of stimulation right to the point of response. Remember how at a routine physical your doctor taps your knee and your lower leg kicks out? Our intestines, believe it or not, are key to how we look and feel, because they are integrally connected via these nerve pathways or meridians to every major organ and to all parts of the body. The impaction of old toxic material in our bowel can affect many other parts of the body, as it can work to send disruptive, weakening reflexes to other parts of the body in many forms, resulting in such ailments as a headache.

If we clear up blocked energy in our intestine, we will be able to free up energy all around the body—including blockages and pain in our shoulders or back. Blood, nerve impulses and lymph can only flow freely when our channels are not blocked. This has implications for our external beauty, as well. For instance, the nasolabial line between the nose and the mouth is directly related to our lung meridian, which also runs through the intestines. This deep wrinkle can get more pronounced the more toxicity we have in our bodies. Likewise, it will start to lighten up naturally as we begin to cleanse by changing our eating habits for the long term.

One of my most delightful results of following the Beauty Detox Solution is that my rather deep "laugh" lines greatly diminished. They weren't really lines just from laughing, after all, but simply toxic blockages in my system!

automatically increase as our bodies will be able to perform digestive and other functions efficiently and with much less effort. Thanks to that renewed energy, we will also lose weight and look years or even decades younger. Our skin will radiate and our hair will grow in with vibrant body and a healthy sheen.

I think you would be surprised to realize how much impacted waste is in our bodies at any given time, continuously poisoning the blood and the entire system to a varying extent. Remember how long and winding our intestinal tract is, and how much space there is to store waste. Since our body is made of spongy tissue through which our blood circulates, this waste can and does permeate our other tissues and organs. Quite a gross and scary thought! But we all need to be aware of this and we all need to cleanse.

Where do these toxins come from? They are the preservatives and chemicals *in* our food, and also food particles that are not properly digested. The improperly digested foods

The Cleaner the Body, the Clearer the Mind

Detoxification is not just about the body. Detoxification also serves to purify the mind, because when our bodies are cleansed, our minds become more clear and we are able to strengthen our focus on what we really want to achieve in our lives. In this clear, clean space, there is no room for chronic negativity, depression, violence, jealousy or anger. We become more naturally magnetic to others, and more at peace with who we really are.

The more internal blockages we have, the less we will feel our absolute best in both our body and mind. Conversely, the cleaner we are, the more energy and focus we have to be able to accomplish our personal, physical and spiritual goals.

There truly is an undeniable connection between our bodies and our minds. Unfortunately, over the last few decades, as medical science has put a large empha-sis on medications and surgery, the emphasis on internal cleansing and the belief in the body's ability to heal itself have virtually disappeared.

The Beauty Detox Solution works to gently loosen up years-old waste in your body and flush it out, along with any past emotions and attachments that may have been "stored" along with it. Ancient Hindu and yogic beliefs teach us that our Manipura chakra, or energy center, is located in our navel and belly area. It is associated with the element of fire and, when blocked, is the place where we can store the emotions of anger and bitterness in our bodies. Clearing out the sludge means we don't have to drag all that "old stuff" around with us anymore. We can live in the present with a much sharper and clearer mind, and discover more joy and happiness.

True Beauty Story

MY CLIENT ALEXIS MOORE IS A SUCCESSFUL, DRIVEN TWENTY-EIGHT-YEAR-OLD WHO has a great job in advertising at a large firm in midtown Manhattan. Like the stereotypical New York young professional, she has a type A personality and lives her life on a very tightly planned schedule—from her prework gym routine to dinner meetings or after-dinner drinks—and packs her weekends with appointments, brunches and get-togethers. She's the kind of girl that wears heels and pearls on Saturday morning and always has perfect makeup and manicured nails. You know who I'm talking about! She approaches her diet from the same controlled perspective. She keeps a food diary and can tell me exactly how many calories and grams of carbs, fat and protein she ate at each meal, as well as during the entire day.

The problem was that even with all that careful counting, Alexis was still a good ten pounds heavier than her ideal weight. For someone very used to controlling outcomes, she was incredibly frustrated with the difficulties she was having with her weight. She did lose weight periodically but always ended up gaining it all back when she didn't follow her closely monitored diet to a T. Of course, it was inevitable that she could not be perfect *all* the time! She wanted to flatten her belly "pooch" and target the fat on her thighs.

Over our sessions I got Alexis to see food as more than just a bunch of numbers. We had an in-depth discussion on how weight loss and energy have everything to do with how well (or poorly) we digest our food. The degree of digestibility and how much certain foods contribute to *sludge* cannot be derived simply from looking at numbers like calorie content.

At first, Alexis was reluctant to let go of her old beliefs, and she wanted to cling to her old foods that were low carb and low calorie (like her daily protein bars) but simultaneously difficult to digest. It was mentally difficult for her to see that she had possibly been doing something wrong for so long. I steered her away from labeling things as "right" or "wrong" by instead using more holistic ways to think about food. How close is the food to its natural state? What sort of process did it undergo to wind up in that package at the grocery store? Our health and weight-loss goals should *always* be looked at from a holistic perspective.

After a few weeks Alexis started to get the hang of evaluating which foods required less energy for digestion, and began to focus her energy on not just counting calories but also on sticking to natural, easily digestible foods. Her energy immediately increased and, as we continued to cleanse, it got higher and higher. She had no problem waking up for her early workouts, and in fact she reported that they got better and even more intense. She trimmed off four pounds the first two weeks, then hit a plateau and fluctuated for the next few weeks. After two months she was down a net of twelve pounds…and she has kept it off now for over a year. Her body looks sleek and trim…hot! Not only did she lose weight, but she eliminated bloat, gas and waste stored in her body.

I see Alexis only occasionally now—when she swoops in wearing her perfectly pressed dress pants and matching tailored shirts, armed with a list of very detailed, specific questions. She has applied that intelligence and energy to going deeper into the Beauty Detox lifestyle. She is vibrant, loving her new body, full of energy, much more lighthearted and, dare I say, more laid-back!

become breeding grounds for "unfriendly" bacteria, yeasts and mold in our body, and the wastes they release are acidic and toxic (for more information on this, see the Alkaline-Acid Principle on page 23).

Only when we cleanse can the energy in our body be distributed to rebuild the beauty and lustrous qualities of our skin and hair, add sheen to our eyes, and firm up and tighten our skin. Even though I have eaten a diet mostly made up of high-quality greens, other vegetables and unprocessed foods for years, I am amazed at how this program continues to work. I am constantly hitting new levels of energy and seeing improvements in my skin and body!

Most diets out there are focused on the number of calories or grams of carbs and protein to consume, yet they make no effort to deduce how efficiently—or not—our system can break down or use any given food. These eating plans do not consider the factor of Beauty Energy and how it is used up in digesting foods that are difficult to break down. You may not even realize which foods are hard to break down, but you will by the end of *The Beauty Detox Solution!*

Calories and grams of carbs and proteins alone do not give a holistic picture of how healthy a food is *within the human body,* how nutrient dense it is or how much fiber it has. Nor do they give us any clues as to the amount of foreign chemicals, preservatives and additives that may be in that given food. That is the very reason that dieting and losing weight have always seemed like such a miserable chore and struggle, a struggle that most of us feel we are losing, along with our energy levels. Don't worry, because you are soon going to learn the *easy* way to lose weight and get your energy back up again!

The high content of enzyme-rich, living foods in the Beauty Detox Solution will help cleanse and unclog the waste from the villi in the intestines so the body can start to absorb nutrients optimally. This creates more Beauty Energy. Weight will come off, and beauty will increase!

We must respect how incredibly powerful our bodies are. Our body has the ability to heal itself, and it will achieve its highest potential if we clear the way for it to do so. We need to clear out all the foreign junk and toxicity. Remember the wheel analogy? We have to get the clogging sludge out of the spokes so we can look and feel our best. Each and every one of us has this potential for natural healing and beauty within us; we just have to understand and work with Beauty Energy to make the most of it.

Building up toxic waste in the body can take many years, even decades, so detoxification on a deeper level is not something that can happen instantly. It should be a gradual, controlled and regulated process . . . and it needs to take place continuously! In fact, detoxification that happens too quickly can be very uncomfortable—we can actually feel or become ill. But we can start to see changes fairly quickly by making important shifts in the foods we are eating, when we eat them, and the order in which we do so.

THE ALKALINE-ACID PRINCIPLE

Perhaps you haven't thought about acid or alkaline measurements since chemistry class in high school. But maintaining the balance of alkalinity and acidity in our bodies and tissues is one of the most important roles of nutrition. We need to understand this principle, as it is key to fighting aging and weight gain.

The balance between alkalinity and acidity is referred to as pH, which stands for "power of hydrogen," and reflects the concentration of hydrogen ions in any given solution. The pH scale ranges from totally acidic at 0.0 to totally alkaline at 14.0, making 7.0 neutral. The higher the pH number of something over 7.0, the more alkaline it is.

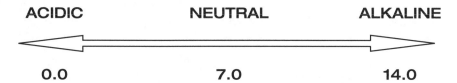

All foods leave either an alkaline or an acidic residue in the bloodstream due to whether they contain more alkaline or more acid minerals. What is important for our health and beauty is the way the foods break down in our body and the *residue* that foods leave. Don't get confused by the fact that the word "acidic" is used to describe the taste or flavor profile of a food. For instance, limes or lemons add an "acid" balance to a recipe, but when *digested,* both leave an alkaline ash in our bodies. It is not helpful to evaluate the pH of a particular food in isolation, because how it breaks down in the body is a whole other story. Dairy milk in isolation has an alkaline pH, but when it is digested it leaves an extremely acidic residue in the body. Digesting animal products also produces acidic compounds.

Different areas of our body have different pH requirements. For instance, our tissues should be slightly alkaline, while our colon should be slightly acidic. When you average all the areas of the body together, the net average would optimally be slightly alkaline. Our ideal blood pH is 7.365,[6] and it must stay within a tight range in order for us to maintain optimal health.[7] Under normal circumstances, and when we are eating a diet rich in alkaline-forming foods, our bodies have no difficulty maintaining this optimal, slightly alkaline pH.

BEAUTY TIP

Overfed, yet Starving for Beauty Nutrients

Another reason we overeat and struggle so much with calorie counting and portion size while still being hungry is that our bodies are not fully absorbing nutrients. Nutrients are absorbed through tiny hairlike villi along the walls of our intestines. We have over seven thousand feet of surface area in our small intestine.

However, if the tiny villi get clogged, we will not feel nourished, no matter how much we eat. The villi are easily clogged by the waste products of foods that our bodies can't metabolize and utilize efficiently, and that also promotes the production of excessive mucus or yeast. Just a few examples of these clogging foods are processed or microwaved foods, canned foods, refined sugars, cow's milk and other dairy products, excessive animal protein and white flour-based foods.

Another way the villi can get clogged is from the excessive growth of yeasts and fungus in the body. In his book *The pH Miracle,* Robert O. Young, Ph.D., explains how yeast and fungus impede nutrient absorption: "They can cover large sections of the membrane lining the inside of the small intestine, displacing probiotics and preventing your body from getting the good stuff out of what you eat. This can leave you starving for vitamins, minerals, and especially protein, regardless of what you actually put in your mouth. I estimate that more than half of adults in the United States are digesting and absorbing less than half of what they eat."[4]

When we aren't absorbing nutrients, our bodies tell us to keep eating, though we have just been fed. Thus begins the utterly deflating and guilt-inducing cycle that most of us are all too familiar with: eating more, even when we know we have just eaten plenty of food and, yes, plenty of calories. I totally understand the frustration and have experienced it myself. *Why am I still hungry when I just ate an eight hundred calorie lunch?*

Raw food nutrition pioneer Dr. Norman Walker writes in depth about the effects of eating processed and devitalized foods. As he explains in *Colon Health:* "If a person has eaten processed, fried and overcooked foods, devitalized starches, sugar and excessive amounts of salt, his colon cannot possibly be efficient, even if he should have a bowel movement two to three times a day!"[5]

In other words, the prevalence of our bowel movements, while very important, does not necessarily indicate how cleansed and toxin free our bodies are. We can still have clogged intestinal villi, as well as impaction and waste matter pushed deep into our bodies, which keeps us from absorbing the nutrients we need.

However, when faced with an acid overload, our bodies have to scramble to find ways to prevent the blood pH from dropping too low, even at the expense of disrupting other tissues, organs and cellular activities in the rest of the body. With the prevalence of too much acid, the body begins to leach alkaline minerals out of the tissues to compensate. The alkaline minerals, like calcium, potassium and magnesium, that we lose in the process also serve many beautifying functions, such as allowing us to have strong, beautiful bones and opening up detoxification pathways in our bodies.

While foods that promote acidity in the body are not all necessarily "bad," those foods must be balanced with alkaline foods. The human body thrives on foods that promote blood alkalinity and help neutralize the acidic waste products of metabolism. Among the most acid-forming of all foods are animal products. When the amount of animal protein ingested increases, so do metabolic acids and wastes.

Research shows the connection between increased animal protein intake and a loss of calcium in the bones, to help neutralize the acid. In 2009 an article in the *New York Times* entitled "Exploring a Low-Acid Diet for Bone Health"[8] discussed how "when the blood becomes even slightly too acid, alkaline calcium compounds—like calcium carbonate, the acid-neutralizer in Tums—are leached from bones to reduce the acidity." The article goes on to state, "The more protein people consume beyond the body's true needs, the more acidic their blood can become and the more alkaline compounds are needed to neutralize the acid.... [I]t does suggest that those at the high end of protein consumption may be better off eating less protein in general and less animal protein in particular and replacing it with more fruits and vegetables."[9]

One study cited in the article analyzed what happened when protein intake (mostly animal based) was doubled from 35 g per day to 78 g per day.[10] The research showed a shocking 50 percent increase in urinary calcium, in other words, calcium that's lost in the body and excreted in the urine. To drive home the very real implications of this study, consider that the average American intake of calcium is between seventy and one hundred grams a day! In 2001 investigations in the Study of Osteoporotic Fractures Research Group at the University of California at San Francisco published the results of a study involving over one thousand women aged sixty-five and older[11] that looked at the proportion of animal to plant protein in their diets over a seven-year period. The women with the lowest ratio of animal-plant protein derived an average of 50 percent of their total protein from animal

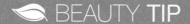

BEAUTY TIP

Cut Out the Soda!

We are well aware that consuming soda loads us up with lots of calories and absolutely no nutrition. But it is not just the calories we are concerned with. Soda (and that includes diet varieties!) is also the most acid-forming of all foods. In fact, soda isn't really a food at all: it is a collection of acidic chemicals, like carbonic acid and phosphoric acid. Soda consumed regularly will demineralize our teeth and rob us of our beauty by eating up the precious minerals that create it.

sources. The study found that women with the highest percentage of animal protein in their diet had 3.7 times more bone fractures and lost bone almost four times faster than the women with the lowest percentage.

An excess of acidity in our bodies is horrifyingly harmful over the short and long term. People that have eaten the standard American diet (SAD) over many years have an excess of acidity in their bodies and this can contribute to poor health, disease, premature death, inflammation, stiffness, tissue degeneration, water retention, bloating and more.

In his book *The pH Miracle,* Dr. Robert Young states, "The pH level of our internal fluids affects every cell in our bodies. The entire metabolic process depends on an alkaline environment. Chronic overacidity corrodes body tissue, and if left unchecked will interrupt all cellular activities and functions, from the beating of your heart to the neural firing of your brain. In other words, acidity interferes with life itself. It is the root of *all* sickness and disease." He goes on to say that "this process of acid waste breakdown and disposal could also be called 'the aging process.'"[12]

Alkaline blood makes for an alkaline body, which promotes health, beauty and longevity, and enables one to fights disease, toxemia and aging. Moreover, weight loss is much easier when our bodies are in an alkaline state. An acidic body tends to hold on to excess weight and makes losing weight a much bigger effort. That's because when overloaded with acid, the eliminative organs, such as the lungs or the kidneys, become overwhelmed and can not remove all the waste. So, much of the toxic, acidic waste gets stored in fatty tissues all over the body, as explained in Chapter 1. The more toxins you have in your body, the more your fat cells expand to store the toxins. Since the body is always trying to protect itself, much of the waste gets pushed away from the vital organs—which is why fat tends to collect in the usual "problem" areas, namely, under the chin, on the upper arms, along the midsection, and along the hips and thighs.

An overly acidic body also greatly diminishes our beauty. Excess acidity can be a major contributing cause of premature aging, along with premature lines and wrinkles; acne; dark under-eye circles; limp, bodiless or otherwise unhealthy hair; and brittle nails. This is why it is important to really understand that these overt symptoms all start with the biochemistry of an acidic body.

In order to make ourselves the healthiest, most youthful and most beautiful we can be, we must support our body's effort to stay at its perfect, slightly alkaline pH by making changes in our diet. We must also become conscious of which foods leave an alkaline residue and which foods leave an acidic residue in our body.

THE 80-20 RATIO

The way to reach our goal to look and feel our best is to strive to eat 80 percent alkaline-forming foods and 20 percent acid-forming foods. The only foods on earth that leave a truly alkaline residue in the body are fresh, ripe fruits and vegetables (except starchy vegetables, like potatoes) and human mother's milk, which is obviously not on the menu for any of us! All other foods are, in varying degrees, acidic.

VERY ALKALINE FOODS	
Ripe fruits	Sprouts
Greens	Other vegetables (excluding starchy varieties)
VERY ACIDIC FOODS	
Alcohol	Drugs, such as antibiotics/steroids
Animal protein	Nicotine
Artificial sweeteners	Processed foods
Caffeine	Refined sugar
Dairy products	Sodas

THE BEAUTY FOOD CIRCLE

We're all pretty familiar with the food pyramid. Though it has been modified, this more modern pyramid still contains the foods that mainstream health institutions have been telling us to eat for decades. The preponderance of the diet is made up of highly refined starches, while milk and meats are a significant part, with their own *separate* categories. No wonder obesity is on the rise and, in varying ways, we are all aging faster and faster.

THE FOOD PYRAMID

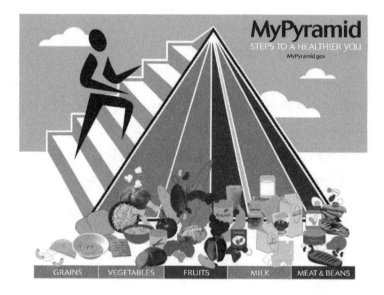

For your Beauty Detox, we're going to think about an entirely different way to balance our diets. We must imagine not a pyramid, but a circle. To look our most beautiful, we need to eat mostly alkalinizing foods, like vegetables and fruits, rounding off the diet with certain whole grains, healthy nuts and limited amounts of oil and animal products.

THE BEAUTY FOOD CIRCLE

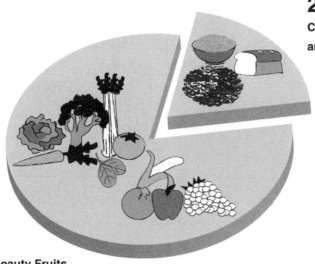

20% Beauty Protein, Carbohydrates, Starches and Fats

80% Beauty Fruits, Greens and Vegetables

When we focus on eating more alkaline foods, it becomes much *simpler* to maintain our weight and improve our health and beauty, without having to get swept into the hype of fixating over one micronutrient or another. Maintaining a high balance of foods that leave an alkaline residue in our bodies will naturally balance our biochemistry. Whole plant foods are easy for our body to digest and will help cleanse our system of toxins so we will get the spectrum of nutrients we need and will absorb our nutrients much better.

You'll see in the proceeding chapters that as we break it down per meal, it's actually a much easier goal to reach the 80% alkaline-forming foods than it might first appear!

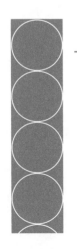

BEAUTY **DETOX** RECAP

- ○ More Energy = More Beauty
- ○ The real cause of aging is acidic sludge in the body, which constantly impedes energy. Ongoing cleansing, which includes consuming cleansing foods, is the way to clean out the sludge.
- ○ Certain foods and combinations of foods digest more easily than others, taking up less Beauty Energy. Freeing up energy from digestion is the single most important way to redirect large amounts of energy to make weight loss efficient and fight aging.

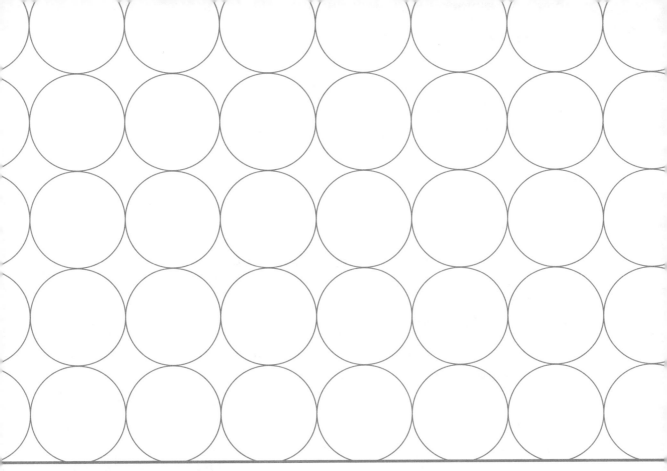

CHAPTER THREE

EATING FOR BEAUTY

A man returned from college with a Ph.D. in making sugar from different fruits. He was asked if sugar could be made from the guava fruit. After some deep thought he said, "I did not study that. It was not in my curriculum." Using common sense was beyond him.

It is not a pumping in from the outside that gives wisdom; it is the power and extent of your inner receptivity that determine how much you can attain of true knowledge, and how rapidly.

—Paramahansa Yogananda

Now that you know that energy creates beauty—clear, youthful skin; lustrous hair; strong nails and a lean body—and the key role digestion plays in Beauty Energy, it's time to start putting it all together. The Beauty Detox Solution goes beyond simply what foods we choose to eat. Beyond incorporating more alkaline foods in your diet, there are ways to actually *eat for beauty*. That's what this chapter is all about! The easy principles in this chapter are the key to maximizing your Beauty Energy, to cleanse the body and make you more beautiful from the inside out.

MORE ENERGY = MORE BEAUTY

EAT ALKALINE FIRST

At each meal, no matter what the whole meal will entail, we always begin by putting an alkaline food *first* in the body—either ripe fruit, raw vegetables or salad. This includes breakfast. Besides ensuring that we consistently load up on raw plant enzymes, practicing this rule will ensure that we get alkaline, water-containing foods in the body at every meal and increase the overall percentage of these foods in our diet.

Do you notice something that these alkaline foods have in common? They contain a great deal of fiber. Fiber acts as a cushion to help slow down glucose absorption in the bloodstream and prevents our blood sugar levels from becoming elevated and erratic. Fiber

What is Fiber?

The Food and Nutrition Board defines dietary fiber as "nondigestible carbohydrates and lignin that are intrinsic and intact in plants."[1] Dietary fiber is found *only* in plant foods and is present in large amounts in fruits, grains, legumes and vegetables. Fiber passes all the way through the small intestine undigested and forms the bulk of our stool. It helps stabilize the body's blood sugar levels, which may help control diabetes. Dietary fiber removes excess cholesterol and hormones, and binds to and deactivates cancer-causing substances.[2]

By working to push toxicity and sludge out of the body on a continual basis, it helps keep the excessive breeding of bad bacteria in check, so our levels of good bacteria stay in the right balance. Fiber also helps us feel full, providing a natural way to fill up on our beautifying plant foods without worrying about restricting or counting calories.

also fills us up and helps diminish our physiological cravings. It is absolutely critical to use this natural way to control portion size. When we fill up first with fresh, natural foods, we can eat in abundance and never feel deprived, since these foods have so much filling fiber and contain so many nutrients.

Fiber also helps keep our digestive tract functioning optimally and keeps us regular, which is critical for our ongoing cleansing efforts. It helps to consistently remove toxins from the body. A report published in the *Journal of the National Cancer Institute* suggested that if one's daily fiber intake was increased by thirteen grams, the risk of colon cancer would decrease by 31 percent.[3] The solution is not to add an isolated fiber supplement, like Metamucil, here and there to a diet filled with foods sorely lacking in crucial dietary fiber. Americans spend $725 million a year on laxatives alone.[4] Something is clearly wrong! Instead, we need to focus on increasing our percentage of high-fiber *foods!* The average American gets only about eight to fourteen grams of fiber a day in his or her diet. On plant-based diets like the Beauty Detox Solution you will get much more—upwards of forty grams of fiber or more![5]

It is easy to have a salad at the start of lunch and dinner at a restaurant or when preparing meals at home. Here are some practical examples of how our Eat Alkaline First principle works in action:

First eat:	Followed by:
Celery sticks	Rolled oat cereal for breakfast
Green salad	Steamed veggies and brown rice at lunch
Green salad	Avocado and veggie sandwich at lunch
Red pepper and carrot sticks	Avocado sushi rolls at lunch
Green salad	Fish and broccoli at dinner

NO MORE CALORIE COUNTING

I have good news. We are not going to be counting calories! Yes, you heard that right: *no more calorie counting!* For generations, people have stayed slim and healthy without ever counting calories. When we look at pictures from the turn of the century to, say, the 1950s, isn't it amazing how relatively slim everyone is? Obesity was not a widespread issue, yet no one counted calories (or anything else, for that matter, like grams of protein or carbs). They also didn't eat all the processed foods and low-fat, low-calorie "diet" foods!

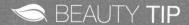

BEAUTY TIP

Be Prepared!

Eat Alkaline First is an important principle to follow. I know we all have busy lives, and it may not always be possible to toss a green salad together before your main meal. So how do you stick to the Beauty Detox while eating out and while traveling? Just plan ahead. For instance, if you are going to a Chinese restaurant for lunch with your coworkers and you know you may have a hard time finding raw vegetables there, prepare ahead of time. Keep some carrots or celery on hand, and eat that within the hour before lunch. When I travel and I know I will be eating less than optimally, I always carry some clementines or carrot sticks that I can eat to make sure I coat my belly first. I also like buying containers of baby spinach, which are easy to grab out of the fridge and knosh on in a pinch when I am preparing something else, or I can also make a very simple salad with it in about thirty seconds.

Calorie counting is a truly modern invention, and it is *not* the only way. Thank goodness, because it is so restrictive and makes for a miserable way to manage our weight! Furthermore, just counting calories won't ensure that you eat foods to promote beauty or help you cleanse your body of aging, acidic sludge. We do want to eat fewer calories in general to maintain our health and weight, but the great news is that we don't have to obsess over it. When you fuel your body with quality, nutritious foods, it happens naturally.

Now, you may be wondering, *Okay, but how much do I eat, then?* Most of us are so out of touch with our true hunger needs, and how much fuel our bodies actually require, that we have no sense of when we're truly hungry or full. As we begin to cleanse the body, our systems will start to optimally absorb nutrients, and we will start feeling full faster. Simultaneously, we will shift into consuming mostly nutrient-dense and fiber-filled foods, which will allow us to get the nutrition with far fewer calories, anyway, whether we are consciously counting or not.

In Part 2, Your Beauty Solution, I provide portion guidelines to get you started. But it is not the purpose of this book to provide you with the minutiae of specific grams of foods and calories you should be eating. These numbers are forever changing depending on which "diet" you are following…not to mention that they're ridiculously confusing! And we all know that calorie counting doesn't work in a consistent way for the long term: there is always that disheartening yo-yo with the scale.

Instead, let's use broader terms for choosing our foods and their quantities—not just numbers. As long as we follow our 80 percent alkaline–20 percent acidic food rule, we will

BEAUTY TIP

Say No to Splenda

Though they have all been approved and declared "safe" for human consumption, there is a lot of controversy and potential health risks associated with artificial sweeteners, which include aspartame (Equal and NutraSweet), saccharin (Sweet 'N Low) and sucralose (Splenda).

Let's start with aspartame, also known as NutraSweet and Equal. As of 1994, 6,888 cases of adverse reactions from aspartame had been reported to the FDA, enough to make up a staggering 75 percent of all nondrug complaints—more than any other food ingredient in the agency's history.[6] Aspartame is an excitotoxin, which is a toxic substance that in high concentrations may stimulate nerve cells so much that they are damaged or killed. It is composed of aspartic acid, methyl ester (which breaks down to formaldehyde and formic acid) and phenylalanine. Those are scary words, right? They point to one thing: that they are acid-forming in the body!

Think aspartame can help you lose weight? Guess again. Despite the fact that it has zero calories, studies have shown that aspartame can in fact *induce* weight gain. Some researchers believe that the two main ingredients in aspartame, phenylalanine and aspartic acid, stimulate the release of insulin and leptin, hormones that instruct our bodies to store fat.[7] One study showed that when we ingest a large amount of phenylalanine, it can drive down our levels of serotonin,[8] which is the neurotransmitter that tells us when we're full. A low level of serotonin can also bring on food cravings.

Saccharin, aka Sweet 'N Low, is no better in this regard. A study at Purdue University's Ingestive Behavior Research Center concluded that consuming foods sweetened with saccharin leads to greater weight gain and body fat than eating the same foods sweetened with sugar.[9]

What about the new popular sweetener sucralose, aka Splenda? Researchers from the Duke University Medical Center published a study in the *Journal of Toxicology and Environmental Health* that showed that sucralose lowered good bacteria in the intestines by 50 percent and contributed to an increase in body weight in lab studies.[10]

The best bet is to avoid all these artificial sweeteners and all products that contain them: there are too many potential health risks. The better choice for a calorie-free sweetener is stevia, which is a natural herb that has been used for hundreds of years in South America and grows naturally in parts of Paraguay and Brazil. It is widely available in the marketplace today. Another good choice is xylitol, a lower calorie, low-glycemic substitute that is a sugar alcohol that occurs naturally in the fibers of many fruits and vegetables. Xylitol is contained in some chewing gums, and it may help reduce cavity-causing bacteria in teeth. If you find that stevia tastes bitter, xylitol may be a better option.

be consuming fewer calories in general, since our concentrated, calorically dense foods will be reduced overall. Have you noticed that there is no nutritional label to read on the side of an apple or a bunch of cilantro? The closer we stick to eating natural, whole and unprocessed foods, which are much easier to digest and free up Beauty Energy, the less we have to worry about counting calories. As we become more alkaline, our bodies will absorb vitamins and minerals, which we'll be getting in abundance, better. We'll also be continually cleaning the sludge out of our wheels, which we now know is the real cause of aging!

Most people try to eat small, restricted portions of low-nutrient foods that have little or no fiber when they try to lose weight. That is why they feel hungry and deprived much of the time. To make things even worse, these diets contribute to aging and create toxins in their bodies. Meat, dairy and refined carbs are so dense in calories and low in fiber and nutrients that it is almost impossible for us to eat them and not consume a huge amount of calories. Or we watch our calories closely and feel miserable all the time, always thinking and obsessing over food! The great news is that on the Beauty Detox Solution, you can eat large amounts of food, but you'll learn to eat truly healthy foods that support cleansing and fill you up with nutrients and fiber. And, no, you'll never have to count another calorie!

BEAUTY FOOD PAIRING

The principle of Beauty Food Pairing is so powerful that it alone can change your entire life. When practiced properly, it will forever improve your beauty and health.

It is *key* that we realize that it is not just what we eat that counts, but what we are able to *use* from what we eat. If we aren't absorbing the vitamins and minerals from that apple we ate this afternoon, it can't possibly make our skin look better, improve our immunity or do anything else to benefit us. We need to pay attention to usable nutrition.

Along those lines, we cannot just read nutritional data on the side of a box to determine the amount of nutrients, protein and vitamins in a particular food and then assume that when we eat that food, we are getting nourished by those nutrients in the exact same amount listed on the label. We have to *digest* foods properly and completely in order to assimilate their nutrients. Many of us aren't digesting our food optimally and therefore are not getting the full amount of nutrition from our foods.

Our bodies are a hot 98.6 degrees, and within them various biochemical reactions take place, all of which must be accounted for. Evaluating a food in isolation is entirely different than evaluating the properties of the food as it is digested and broken down in our bodies. Because our bodies run at such a hot temperature, the longer a food stays in our bodies, the greater the chance that residue from the food will bake and lodge in our bodies and contribute to *sludge*.

Beauty Food Pairing, which incorporates the hard and true tenets of classic food combining—which foods are best to eat together, and which combinations should be avoided at all costs—has a direct impact on our body's ability to break down foods easily and properly, thereby *saving* us large amounts of energy. Remember:

MORE ENERGY = MORE BEAUTY

Beauty Food Pairing is a concept that is not often discussed in our modern world and one that most mainstream health practitioners would dismiss, arguing that we are omnivores and should be able to digest everything we eat. After all, each and every day most of us put a whole lot of different heavy foods into our bodies, all mixed together at the same time. This is an incredibly heavy digestive burden that we are asking our bodies to bear. No, we aren't dying on the spot…but what is the long-term cost? As a society we are getting *fat* and aging *fast.* That is not optimal! If we want to look and feel excellent, we need to do something different and better than what we've been doing. This something different involves *optimizing* digestion, to free up lots of Beauty Energy!

Beauty Food Pairing is not even widely practiced in what are considered progressive nutrition movements, such as the raw food movement. I actually think a lot of raw foodists would benefit from applying this knowledge, as I have many clients that eat all or mostly raw foods and still struggle with their weight and energy levels (and don't always look that great). And it is no wonder. There are many energy-zapping, poorly combined raw food dishes.

Beauty Food Pairing is also something I, too, ignored for years. My health and energy improved tremendously when I shifted into eating more raw plant foods, but at some point I hit a plateau. I still had what seemed to be a "coating" over my muscles and abdomen…and I wanted to drop those last five pounds. Plus, I still regularly felt bloating and gassiness, and I knew my skin could be smoother and brighter. And what was up with those zits that still cropped up periodically? Wasn't a mostly raw, plant-based diet supposed to be so "clean" that it would get rid of all those issues? Something was off.

I had heard about food combining, but like most raw foodists and, well, most other people who have even *heard* of it, I had deliberately chosen to ignore it. My very first reaction was, "I've already cut so many foods out of my diet. On top of that, this sounds like it will make things more restrictive!" Still, I decided to give it a real go and used my own diet as the experiment.

And guess what? *I was astonished at how well it worked!* As they say, the proof is in the pudding. Nothing resonates as truth like personal experience. My energy skyrocketed. I shed another five pounds, which I have been easily able to keep off. My skin became glowing, any gassiness I had disappeared and my body looked much more toned—without doing anything else differently! This was especially true for my upper arms, where I had always longed for defined muscles. I had reached a whole new level of health and beauty.

True Beauty Story

AVA BLOOMQUIST, ONE OF MY CLIENTS, IS SIXTY-TWO YEARS OLD AND A HARD-CORE Brooklynite. She is a skeptic and always makes me laugh with her funny, squinting facial expressions when I tell her something she doesn't believe—at least at first. When I first told her we weren't going to be counting calories, she displayed more than her usual level of disbelief. "How do I know how much I'm supposed to eat when you're not around?" she exclaimed. "I've been counting calories for decades." I teased her, "And it hasn't really worked out so great, has it?" She was really nervous about eating too much, since one of her main goals was to lose thirty pounds.

She started the Beauty Detox and was soon delighted to realize she was losing weight without counting calories. We focused on starting each meal with raw veggies and worked to increase her percentage of them. Instead of her constant deluge of snacks, we added the Glowing Green Smoothie (discussed later) at breakfast, followed by some gluten-free crackers, which she loves. Lunch was usually a salad with veggies and an avocado, followed by some kind of vegetarian soup.

Her body has become more balanced, and her cravings have started to diminish. We have been working together six months, and she has lost over twenty-five pounds! She is losing weight steadily, and most importantly, she is keeping it off long term. In the past, when counting calories and following other diet programs, she always gained the weight back soon after losing it, but not this time. She is smiling more than squinting at me these days!

Now, after practicing proper Beauty Food Pairing for years, if I go back and eat a miscombined meal, I bloat out like an overexpanded balloon and feel exhausted. My body has become quite the Beauty Food Pairing "snob," accustomed to having the best combinations of foods to digest. I was in L.A. recently and went to visit a raw food café, where the owner made me a raw dish that was a mishmash of fresh fruit, dried fruit, nuts and soaked grains. After eating a small bowl of it, I became so uncomfortable and gassy that I excused myself to go to the car for a moment to relax and proceeded to fall asleep for about twenty minutes! Everyone wondered what had happened to me. That's not how I want to be feeling after I eat!

Since then, I have shared Beauty Food Pairing with my clients, and it has helped them tremendously. Try it for *yourself* and say goodbye to bloating, watch the pounds drop and see how your skin becomes even more radiant. And by the way, it is *not* restrictive at all, once you get the hang of it!

Beauty Food Pairing works, and it works amazingly well. The concept is applicable and highly beneficial to *all* diets, whether you eat meat, fish, mostly raw plant foods or are a full-fledged vegan. Though Beauty Food Pairing is seldom discussed in the Western nutrition world and your doctor might shrug it off, that in no way makes it less valid. Remember that the average doctor might spend only about two weeks studying nutrition in medical school—or less. One published study suggests that only about 25 percent of medical schools require training in the medical nutrition sciences,[11] and when medical schools do offer nutrition electives, there are generally low enrollments. It is simply not doctors' area of expertise—even though they have lots of training in many other areas. Therefore, we should go to the experts on nutrition when we want answers, and there are those that have studied the principles of food combining for decades.

HOW BEAUTY FOOD PAIRING WORKS

In order to lose weight and look your most beautiful, you must free up energy from digestion. In addition to the foods we eat, we can increase or decrease Beauty Energy by the order in which we eat foods and the choice of foods we eat together. Remember:

MORE ENERGY = MORE BEAUTY

One of the biggest ailments of the Western world is a chronic lack of energy. A lack of energy can lead to a viciously frustrating cycle of overeating, constant snacking, and reaching for sugary, caffeinated beverages, all in an attempt to feel more energetic and not have to struggle through the day. And, as you now know, a lack of energy makes you hold on to excess weight and look less beautiful. And why are we so tired? Because we're not combining our foods properly.

Beauty Food Pairing is based on the science of how food digests *optimally* in the body. Different foods digest with different enzymes, and some call for more acidic or more alkaline environments. Dr. Herbert M. Shelton is generally considered the foremost expert on food combining. He spent years studying the way digestive enzymes work to help break down foods, the primary basis for Beauty Food Pairing. As Dr. Shelton explains, "Every student of physiology is well aware that the digestive enzymes have certain well-defined limitations and that different digestive juices are secreted for use in digesting different kinds of food substances."[12]

True Beauty Story

MY CLIENT MELANIE LEE IS THIRTY-NINE YEARS OLD AND TRAVELS CONSTANTLY FOR her finance-related job. She has a lot of pressure on her to perform and close deals and have successful meetings with clients, and all the traveling adds to her stress. One of the few things that gives her a sense of stability and comfort is her favorite foods that she likes to fall back on, some of which she knows she can usually get in airport terminals and in the first-class section of planes.

We had to work out a food plan for her quickly because she was on a downward spiral. She was incredibly stressed, had super-low energy and a lot of bloating issues, and her skin was breaking out and looked horrible. It was not a great time to make new food changes, but the one thing I saw from glancing at her diet was that we could easily work out a new food plan by changing only the *order and combination* of the foods she was eating, not the foods themselves.

I talked to Melanie about a month later and she was thrilled! She was feeling much more energetic, and just from changing her food combinations, she had lost seven pounds—mostly old waste trapped in her body! Now she is truly her perfect weight and her body looks much sleeker. Her energy is super high, and she is so happy that she did not have to give up all her comfort foods to look and feel as good as she does now.

During her thirty-five years of study in nutrition, Dr. Ann Wigmore, creator of the Living Foods Lifestyle, adamantly believed that "proper food combining is important for good health."[13] I took classes on food combining as part of the programs I attended at her institute in Rincón, Puerto Rico. The principles of food combining are also taught at the Hippocrates Health Institute in West Palm Beach, Florida, a prestigious and world-famous natural healing center. Ivan Pavlov (well-known for his research about dogs and conditioned response) outlined the fundamental concepts of proper food combining in his book *The Work of the Digestive Glands,* first published in 1902. And Dr. Philip Norman, a prominent gastroenterologist and professor in his time, wrote about the principles of food combining and its key benefits, namely, making digestion more effective.[14] The popular 1980s book *Fit for Life,* by natural hygienists Harvey and Marilyn Diamond, also advocates food combining, as do many of Dr. Norman Walker's writings.[15]

So how does Beauty Food Pairing work? Let's get right into it!

BEAUTY RULE #1: OUR BODIES CAN PROPERLY DIGEST ONLY ONE CONCENTRATED, NON-WATER-CONTAINING FOOD AT A TIME.

To understand this rule, it helps to think back to the gorilla in Chapter 1. That gorilla eats a fairly simple diet, with alkaline, water-based foods at the heart of it: fresh fruits and vegetables. The more simple our meals are, the better digestion will be.

One way to think about eating simpler foods is to classify foods as concentrated and non-concentrated. Concentrated foods are foods that do not contain any water. They include all proteins and starches. Non-concentrated foods are water-containing foods. The only truly non-concentrated foods are ripe fruits and non-starch vegetables.

Non-Concentrated Foods	Concentrated Foods
Ripe fruit	All starches (grains, starchy vegetables, breads, etc.)
Non-starch vegetables	All proteins (fish, chicken, meat, seeds, nuts, etc.)

To sum up, anything that is not a fruit or a non-starch vegetable is a concentrated food. Anything come to mind? Yes, I thought so! A few random examples are nuts, bagels, yogurt, toast, scrambled eggs, ice cream, flax crackers, peanut butter, lobster, etc.

The stomach secretes different kinds of juices when we eat different kinds of foods. Non-concentrated foods are much simpler for the body to digest than concentrated foods. We can handle most concentrated foods pretty well, but we can eat only one *type* at a time in order to maximize digestion. It is a huge Beauty Energy drain to ask our bodies to eat two different types of concentrated foods at one time. The two main types of concentrated foods that we will discuss first are starches and proteins, which leads us to the next Beauty Rule....

BEAUTY RULE #2: PROTEINS AND STARCHES DON'T MIX.

As you read these words, perhaps some favorite or long-accepted food combinations pop into your head: bagels and cream cheese, turkey sandwiches, eggs with toast, sushi rolls, grilled fish and wild rice, filet mignon and potatoes au gratin, chicken pad thai.... Yep, these are all improper food combinations.

I hate to be the bearer of bad news, except that I know that it is in your best interest to be aware of this now. Forget the past, and forget all the years of improperly combining foods. When we have new information, we change! And, remember Melanie's story—we don't have to say goodbye to our favorite comfort foods. *We can eat them in moderation, but just not all of them at the same time.*

To understand why protein and starches don't pair well together, you have to understand how these concentrated foods digest.

PROTEIN: In the stomach a concentrated protein requires an *acidic* environment to be broken down, an environment that includes hydrochloric acid and an enzyme called pepsin.

Examples of Protein:

Chicken	Fish and seafood	Protein powders of all kinds, including whey, soy, hemp, etc.
Dairy (except butter)	Meat	Seeds and nuts
Egg		

STARCH: The breakdown of starch starts with an enzyme called ptyalin (salivary amylase), which can efficiently act only in an *alkaline* medium.

Examples of Starch:

Crackers	Pasta	Cereal	Bread
Grains (rice, wheat, quinoa, millet, etc.)			
Starchy vegetables (yams, sweet potatoes, white potatoes)			

Now think back to high school chemistry class. What happens when an acid and an alkaline are put together? *They neutralize each other.* To use the words of Dr. Norman Walker, eating carbohydrates with protein at the same time results in a "serious chemical situation to contend with."[16]

Since the food is not breaking down naturally, what do our poor glands do next? Our stomach has to secrete more digestive juices to try to break down the food, but because there are still opposing digestive enzymes at work, they are neutralized again and again. The digestion of the carbohydrates is interfered with by the presence of the acidic digestive juices, and at the same time the proteins are prevented from digesting properly or completely in the presence of the alkaline digestive juices.

This inefficient digestive process takes hours, costing us copious amounts of Beauty Energy. We immediately get *tired* after eating because all our energy is going right into our bellies. It is analogous to a nice Ferrari stuck in the mud with its wheels spinning. No matter how much we jam on the accelerator, the car stays right where it is, just spinning and wasting even more energy. We may experience gassiness, bloating and/or heartburn. Since we get tired pretty quickly after this ill-combined meal, this leads to a groggy afternoon with multiple trips to the company coffee machine or Starbucks, or an uninspired evening in front of the TV. Sound familiar?

Even with the huge sacrifice of so much of our Beauty Energy, the food in this poorly combined meal is never 100 percent digested. There is a major problem with all this: The longer a food stays in the 98.6-degree body, and the slower it moves through our digestive system, the greater chance it has to become toxic residue as it bakes in our body at this high temperature. In contrast, the faster a food passes through our system, providing us with adequate nutrition and then exiting, the healthier it is.

Because of these long hours of stasis in our hot bellies, much of the protein in the stomach will become putrefied (rotten), and much of the carbohydrates will become fermented.[17] Now we are dealing with literally rotting matter. Much of the nutrition within those foods is lost, while we are exhausted because the body wastes incredible amounts of energy trying to break the food down.

Putrefied protein and fermented carbohydrates are unusable by the body and will not contribute to healthy, beautiful cell structure. We do not derive any value from foods that are improperly digested in this manner. As Dr. Norman Walker aptly puts it, "The greatest friends of old age are fermentation and putrefaction. Both of these are natural processes of disintegration. That is why they speed up the aging of people."[18]

ROTTEN STARCH + ROTTEN PROTEIN = MORE TOXIC SLUDGE IN OUR BODIES

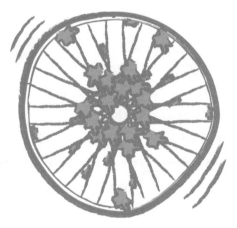

Poor food pairing adds more toxic sludge to the wheel.

A large component of this constantly amassing sludge comes from fermented and putrefied material, which is built up largely from improper Beauty Food Pairings. It is indeed muddying up our natural beauty, dulling our radiance and contributing to our *getting old!* Sludge slows down our systems and makes us pack on the pounds, especially around our belly area, no matter how relatively few calories we consume.

When the food is finally pushed out of the stomach, where it has been for hours, it still has to navigate through about thirty feet of winding intestinal tract! The food could take some twenty to forty hours (or more) to get through the intestines.[19] That, my friends, is what we call a serious Beauty Energy *drain*. Besides that, we just don't get the most nutrition from our food when we don't adhere to the laws of Beauty Food Pairing.

IMPROPER BEAUTY FOOD PAIRINGS:

Skinless chicken breast with potatoes	Lean turkey meat on whole-wheat bread
Tuna or salmon sushi rolls	Egg white omelet with whole-grain toast
Grilled or baked fish over wild rice	Low-fat cream cheese on a bagel

We have been led to believe these combinations are okay—even healthy!—because they are low in fat. But they are in fact aging, slow-digesting foods that when combined contribute to the sludge in our bodies.

Not combining proteins and starches at the same meal will optimize the amount of nutrients you can extract from foods and will free up a lot of energy. Instead of having an energy deficit, you will have an energy surplus. You will have the energy to kick butt at work, get through a whole afternoon without needing an extra cup of coffee, get a whole lot more done around the house and literally run laps around your roommate, spouse or your kids.

BEAUTY TIP

You Don't Have to Be Perfect All the Time

Of course, the reality is that sometimes we are going to miscombine foods. Sometimes, especially in the beginning and when we are transitioning, we simply *must* have our favorite sushi rolls or a tuna fish sandwich from our favorite deli or (gasp!) a hamburger. We are not expected to be perfect all the time. The occasional miscombining is okay, as long as we realize it will take us a step back and not a step forward. As you start Beauty Food Pairing, you will love how much more energy you have and how much better you feel, so you'll want to avoid miscombining naturally.

If you are going to miscombine, do it later on in the day, ideally at dinner. (We'll discuss more on that in Light to Heavy.) On these occasions, you should balance your foods like a seesaw. On one side of the seesaw are foods that are optimal for your health: salads, vegetables, fruit. On the other side are concentrated, miscombined foods. If you eat those miscombined foods, you have to balance them out with the optimal foods—the heavier the miscombined foods, the more optimal foods you pile on to keep the seesaw balanced for beauty. If you're going to have a heavy, miscombined dinner, start with an oil-free green salad. The salad will help neutralize some of the digestive distress the improperly combined meal creates. It will also coat the stomach with fiber and help the heavier foods digest better—while ensuring you reduce your portion sizes of them!

Okay, now for the good news! Remember when I said you wouldn't have to give up all your favorite foods and ban them forever? The best part is, we can still eat the foods we like, just *not all at the same time!* The general rule is to wait three to four hours before eating one concentrated food before eating another so we have time to clear the first food out of our bellies first. Then, we are home free.

BEAUTY RULE #3: VEGETABLES ARE NEUTRAL.

Vegetables are wonderful alkaline, non-concentrated foods. They are simple for our body to digest and are considered absolutely neutral. If you love roasted chicken or steamed tilapia fish, eat it along with some steamed vegetables and a raw green salad. If you are in the mood for a starchy dish, maybe some pasta salad or a baked yam, eat it with some vegetables.

BEAUTY RULE #4: MIXING TWO STARCHES IS OKAY.

Even though starches are concentrated foods, they aren't as complicated to digest as protein. While simple meals are always best, two different starches are okay to eat at once.

BEAUTY RULE #5: MIXING TWO DIFFERENT TYPES OF ANIMAL PROTEIN IS NOT OKAY.

Proteins as a whole are the hardest food group to break down. Proteins are comprised of complex chains of amino acids, each with a very different character and chemical makeup. Our bodies must break down protein into amino acids in order to digest or assimilate them. Since the body has to concentrate so much energy on breaking down each protein, only one protein at a time should be consumed. Otherwise, the proteins will not fully and efficiently digest, and they will putrefy in the digestive tract.

Animal proteins are much more complex and difficult to break down than plant proteins, which include seeds, nuts and sea algae, and this means this rule is really only applicable to animal proteins. You can mix plant proteins without a problem, so, for example, having seeds and nuts together is fine. But surf and turf, eggs with ham, or an appetizer containing fish followed by a chicken main dish are all bad combinations. Two kinds of fish or two kinds of poultry eaten together at the same meal are okay, but remember to keep meals as simple as possible to preserve Beauty Energy.

BEAUTY RULE #6: FATS SHOULD BE EATEN MODERATELY WITH PROTEIN (ANIMAL AND PLANT) BUT ARE OKAY TO EAT WITH CARBOHYDRATES.

Fat mixes well with starches but has somewhat of an inhibiting effect on the digestion of protein.[20] You can pair minimal amounts of fat with protein, but it is best not to eat a *large* amount of fat with any protein. Even if you are eating an all-raw meal, it is best not to mix a lot of nuts (protein) together with a whole avocado (fat)! This could prevent efficient weight loss. A plentiful supply of green vegetables can be used to counteract the interaction between a moderate amount of protein and raw fat. For instance, if you are having a piece of fish over a nice green salad, it is okay to have a little oil on the salad, but go easy on it and eat up a good portion of the alkaline greens first. But if weight loss is truly the goal, it would be best to skip the oil altogether and let the protein digest perfectly on its own!

BEAUTY RULE #7: FRUIT SHOULD BE EATEN ONLY ON AN EMPTY STOMACH.

The first time I talked publicly about how to eat fruit was on one of my segments for *Good Morning America*. Millions of people watched the show, and dozens of people wrote to me

True Beauty Story

MY CLIENT CLARA EVANS IS A FORTY-SIX-YEAR-OLD FROM MICHIGAN, AND WE DO OUR nutritional consultations over the phone. She was concerned about a lack of energy and motivation in life in general. She has two teenage sons and a husband who works in construction and does not consider a meal to be "real" if there's not a hunk of meat on the plate. She does not have the money or the time to make separate meals for herself and her boys every night.

Other than adding some veggie sticks to her mornings, we changed only the *combination* and order of the foods she was already eating. She did *not* have to increase her food budget or slave away making double meals. Within weeks Clara reported back that she had lost eight pounds, felt completely energized during the day and was sleeping much better! She even reported that her eyes were looking brighter and one of her neighbors asked her if she had had Botox injections, since her face had already started to look fresh and years younger!

Beauty Food Pairing Cheat Sheet

Starches DO mix with vegetables

Proteins DO mix with vegetables

Proteins and starches DO NOT mix

Different starches DO mix

Different proteins DO NOT mix

Fats DO NOT mix well with protein; pair moderately

Fats DO mix with starches

Fruits should be eaten on an empty stomach

Fruit DOES mix with raw greens (except melons)

afterward, fascinated to know more about how to properly eat fruit. It's very simple: eat fruit on an empty stomach.

Fruit is considered the most divine and pure food on the planet. Fruit increases our vitality and delivers key vitamins, minerals and pure, filtered water into our bodies. However, *when* we eat fruit is key. So, you may think you're opting for the healthy choice when you go for the fruit salad for dessert, but you're just going to make digestive trouble! Fruit breaks down the quickest of all foods; it is out of the stomach in twenty to thirty minutes. If it has to sit on top of foods that take longer to digest and leave the stomach, namely, concentrated foods like starch and protein, it will ferment and acidify the whole meal.

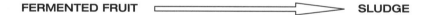

FERMENTED FRUIT ⟹ SLUDGE

Fruits (except for melons) combine well with fresh, raw greens. Fruits and greens form the perfect pair in the Glowing Green Smoothie and the Glowing Green Juice, which we'll discuss later on in the Beauty Minerals section.

◖ BEAUTY TIP

Good Beauty Food Pairing Dishes

Even if you aren't yet eating according to the Beauty Food Circle, you can still benefit from Beauty Food Pairing. These examples are to show that *all* of us, no matter what kind of diet we are currently eating, can start practicing Beauty Food Pairing right now.

- Avocado sushi rolls
- Grilled fish on a bed of mesclun greens
- Guacamole with salad and corn chips
- Steak with slightly sautéed spinach
- Bagel with organic butter
- Apple, followed by scrambled eggs twenty minutes later
- Baked chicken with broccoli
- Pasta primavera

I am *so* excited for you to try out Beauty Food Pairing and experience the spectacular results for yourself. I have done my best to present to you the research and science that are out there to support Beauty Food Pairing, but remember that the best study out there in regards to this principle is to try it out for yourself! In a short amount of time you will see how well it truly does work. And isn't that the most important thing? There will always be conflicting and confusing reports of "scientific evidence," or lack thereof, with regard to nutritional information. *But if you try something for yourself, and you see that it truly helps you lose weight and look and feel amazing—the way Beauty Food Pairing does—who cares about all the "noise" out there?* Use it to your personal beauty and health advantage.

Now you have the basic guidelines to free up major amounts of Beauty Energy and greatly promote digestion, which you probably weren't even aware you were hindering before. If this seems confusing to you, don't worry, because the meal plans in Part 2, Your Beauty Solution, are all de-

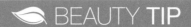

BEAUTY TIP

How Water Fits In

We've all heard how important it is to stay hydrated, and we all need pure, filtered, non-tap water. However, when we start eating the Beauty Detox way, we will be getting water from lots of water-containing fruits and vegetables, so we may not all need to adhere to the general recommendation of eight full glasses of water a day. Individualize and drink the amount your body needs.

It is important to drink water when we wake up and throughout the morning so we start our day hydrated. Just by ensuring we are hydrated like this will give us more energy.

Drink significant quantities of water at least half an hour *before* your meals or an hour *following* meals. During mealtimes, we must drink as little as possible. Too much liquid with meals dilutes our digestive juices and delays digestion considerably. What happens when digestion is delayed? It contributes to the dreaded sludge by increasing the chances that putrefaction and fermentation will occur.

Get in the habit of squeezing some liver-supporting, vitamin C-filled lemon in your water for an added benefit!

signed with Beauty Food Pairing in mind. You can also photocopy the Beauty Food Pairing Cheat Sheet and keep it at your desk or in your purse.

Beauty Food Pairing alone will help you lose weight, look younger and more alive, and have much more energy!

MORE ENERGY = MORE BEAUTY

Remember, Beauty Food Pairing is not an all-or-nothing endeavor. It does not mean that if you improperly combine foods at a meal, you are doomed. *Combine well where you can, and proceed at your own pace.* The more motivated you are and the more you practice proper food combining, the better your results will be. Beauty Food Pairing alone will do wonders to help reduce the girth of our bellies. It is not just excess weight pushing our bellies out, but also distension from gas pressure and bloating created from poor food combinations.

Think about all the energy you've spent trying to digest hard-to-break-down food combinations. All that energy can now be redirected toward detoxifying your body and subsequently losing weight, building strong nails, growing healthy, thick hair and creating glowing skin.

BEAUTY TIP

Nipping Acne in the Bud

Our skin is our biggest organ, and it is also our largest detoxifying organ. We expel pounds of waste and toxins through our skin daily. When our skin erupts into chronic acne, the allopathic approach is to assume something is clogging the skin's surface locally and to use prescription topical creams. The issue with that, as with all medications, is that piling them on or in the body merely suppresses the symptoms. They don't get to the root cause.

I am a huge advocate of using the right products on your skin, but if you are using the right cleansers and other good, non-clogging products and you *still* have an acne issue that is affecting your self-esteem and you are considering trying a prescription medication or even antibiotics, then there is probably a much deeper problem going on.

Our skin is like an external monitor that provides us with information about the internal state of our liver, our blood and our colon. Acne is often a symptom of something happening inside, so we need to treat the *cause* and not just the effect.

When our skin has to pour out so many toxins that it erupts into acne, that is a red flag that toxicity, bacteria, and/or yeast is overwhelming the body. Usually, our liver eliminates toxins and impurities by pushing them into the colon. But this works only when the colon is clean and functioning optimally. If the colon is clogged and backed up (which can happen on a deeper level even if we are regularly going to the bathroom), and/or if our bodies have become overly acidic and a fertile breeding ground for unfriendly bacteria, our liver will get clogged and backed up, and toxins will be pushed out through the skin…and then the acne shows up!

We will uncover how you can cleanse the body internally with nature's strongest food scrubs and probiotics to kick your acne out once and for all. And when acne crops up, you will know what that indicates and how to eat and cleanse your way back to clear skin.

EAT LIGHT TO HEAVY

Now that we've learned about Beauty Food Pairing together, here is the next piece that we need to put the methodology into practice: Light to Heavy.[21] It is not just *what* we eat that matters, or even just the combination, but also the *order* in which we eat our food.

Like Beauty Food Pairing, Light to Heavy is designed to make food move as quickly as possible through our bodies. As we've been stressing throughout the book, it is all about speed: we want nutrients in the food to absorb quickly and the rest of the food to pass through. Speed reduces fermentation, putrefaction, gassiness and bloating—not to mention wasted Beauty Energy…all the things that contribute to aging.

SPEED IS POSSIBLE ONLY IF WE AVOID A TRAFFIC JAM

Imagine if there was a Porsche, a Land Rover, and a sixteen-wheel truck on the highway, and you were the traffic marshal that had all the authority to position each vehicle along the highway to avoid traffic. How would you position the vehicles so that traffic would move efficiently down the highway?

ROUTE BEAUTY

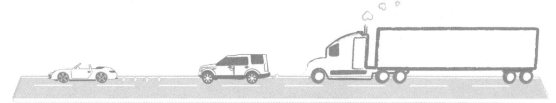

In this order, all vehicles can speed along and traffic is avoided! But what happens when we switch the order?

TRAFFIC JAM

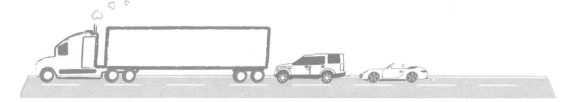

Under this second scenario, the highway is all backed up, and we have caused a traffic jam. The Porsche is stuck in the back, spinning its wheels. How does this apply to our food?

We've already discussed that the longer a food stays in our system, the longer it has to putrefy and ferment.

Therefore, we need to be aware of how fast foods move in general, and eat the lightest food items first, ending with the heaviest food items, to keep the food passing through as fast as possible.

The lightest foods move the fastest through the stomach and the heaviest ones move the slowest. Fruit passes through the stomach in about twenty to thirty minutes, with the exception of the banana, which takes about forty-five minutes. Starches remain in the stomach a few hours, and proteins even longer, as they are the slowest moving and take the most work to break down. That is why it is generally recommended to wait three to four hours before switching to a different food group.

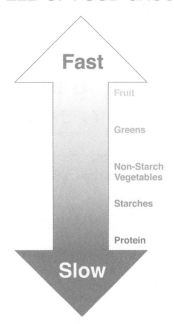

SPEED OF FOOD GROUP

Fast

Fruit

Greens

Non-Starch Vegetables

Starches

Protein

Slow

What if the three foods we were going to eat were fruit, salad and fish? Based on our Speed of Food Group chart, this would be the order in which we would have to eat these foods to avoid a traffic jam in our stomachs:

ROUTE BEAUTY

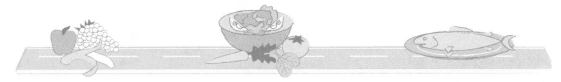

In this order, all food can speed along our digestive tract and a traffic jam is avoided! We would wait at least twenty minutes after eating the fruit to eat the rest of the meal to let the fast-moving fruit get through. The salad could be eaten right before the fish so we load up on water, fiber and lots of plant nutrients first. With greens and non-starch vegetables we do *not* have to wait twenty minutes to eat other foods, the way we do with fruit. But now let's see what happens when we switch the order:

TRAFFIC JAM

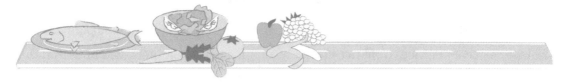

In this scenario, we are all backed up. The protein in the fish is sitting in our stomach, blocking lighter foods from passing through. Having fruit for dessert has created a bloating internal mess! The fruit is fermented by the time it reaches the intestines, where we need to absorb its nutrients. But now, there are barely any nutrients left to absorb.

For your Beauty Detox, breakfast starts with fruit, veggie sticks or a green drink, even if heavier foods follow while we are transitioning. Juice is the purest food of all, since it is not a solid food but a liquid, and should always be consumed on an empty stomach so that it can be absorbed into the body first. If we eat some toast or hot cereal after the fruit, veggie or green drink, those heavier foods will not block the flow of the lighter foods through our system. The same concept holds true at all meals of the day. Since salad is faster moving than a roasted chicken and packed with good dietary fiber, we should eat a good portion of the salad *first* to help increase the speed of the entire meal through our bodies. Eating the chicken first will prevent the salad from digesting easily and will cause a major traffic jam. Dr. Ann Wigmore recommends that we "eat raw food at a meal before any cooked food. Otherwise the cooked food eaten holds up the digestion of the raw and the latter can ferment, causing uncomfortable gas."

Eating Light to Heavy at each meal will prevent any backup in our system and will keep us from squandering Beauty Energy. We must avoid a traffic jam from occurring in our stomach at all costs. We learned how this can happen in the last section with improper Beauty Food Pairing—it can also happen with eating *heavy to light*. The disastrous consequences from eating, say, fruit after a protein meal, or a green drink after an avocado sandwich, include fermentation, putrefaction, bloat, gas and weight gain. It will also rob us of our Beauty Energy.

MORE ENERGY = MORE BEAUTY
SLOW PASSAGE OF FOOD = FAST AGING

YOUR BEAUTY FOOD PLAN

The Light-to-Heavy principle has an important bearing on our overall food plan. Most of us have been conditioned to eat in a certain way, and it has been ingrained in us that this way is the "healthiest." Let's take a close reexamination.

Traditional Food Plan

BREAKFAST
Popular Belief: Breakfast is the most important meal of the day.

LUNCH
Popular Belief: Lunch should be the heaviest meal of the day so we have time to burn off the calories.

DINNER
Popular Belief: Don't eat as much at dinner, because you won't have time to work off the food.

SNACKS
Popular Belief: Eat little mini meals throughout the day, every few hours, to keep the metabolism running high.

We can see that eating according to this kind of schedule will produce significant backup:

ROUTE BEAUTY

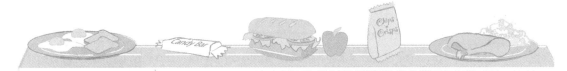

There are multiple traffic jams along the road when we eat this way. Our bodies do not have time to fully digest one food or meal before a new one is consumed. Bad news!

It's clear that the old food plan doesn't work. We have to think about breakfast, lunch and dinner in an entirely new way.

BREAKFAST

We've all been told that breakfast is the most important meal of the day. According to this old belief, we need to stock up at this important first meal in order to supply ourselves with energy to get going. Many of us eat breakfast first thing upon waking up in the morning or soon after. Some of us may even eat early "for energy" when we are not yet hungry.

The first new rule about breakfast is this: *We will never eat when we are not hungry.* If our body is not telling us we are hungry, it is also telling us that it certainly doesn't need any food.

What we do in the morning is critical for achieving our goals. When you wake up in the morning, you have a fresh start. You have not put any *new* food in your body since the evening before, so your body will go to work eliminating and cleaning out what is already in the system. For many of us, this is the *only* time when our body's energy is not consumed in digesting something but can instead be directed to actually cleansing. In the morning we may wake up with some pungent body odors, bad breath, a coated tongue, sleep in our eyes, etc. We can be downright stinky! All these odors and substances coming up to the

True Beauty Story

MEGAN PARKER, AGE THIRTY-THREE, IS A CLIENT OF MINE THAT HAS BATTLED ACNE for most of her life. She had been going to the dermatologist for years and had tried everything, from oral antibiotics to prescription creams and even chemical peels. She had used so many products on her skin that there were patches of redness, flakiness and dryness…but underneath were still confidence-killing fields of enormous cystic pimples and whiteheads. She was extremely frustrated and did not understand why she had tried every professional remedy and every skin-care product out there and still had had no good results.

Instead of targeting the outward symptom of the acne, I looked at the underlying causes in her diet. Her diet was loaded with low-fat dairy products, gluten, soy and other clogging foods. We cut out these foods and created a dietary program for her that included cleansing and detoxifying foods with lots of enzymes and fiber to help slough away the internal sludge that had been causing a backup in her system for years.

We also incorporated some other cleansing techniques, which included ingesting a daily probiotic. Within a few weeks her skin became dramatically clearer, and even her old acne scars seemed to be fading away. After two months she stopped taking her oral medication. Today she still uses good skin-care products for acne-prone skin and a prescription acne cream a few times a week. However, now her skin is beautiful and clear, with no more cystic acne. She is in awe that the secret to beautiful skin really lies in the intestine and liver!

surface are the result of various forms of cleansing that our body has employed throughout the night in order to eliminate toxins.

Morning time until noon is key for cleansing and achieving complete elimination. We learned from our Beauty Energy principle that we have only so much energy to use, and that it must be carefully preserved. The second we start eating again in the day, we shut off the body's cleansing mechanism and our energy has to be directed to digestion. Morning provides us with a literal clean start to let the body root out toxins and eliminate waste. When I say eliminate, yes, I *do* mean go to the bathroom! Above all, we do not want to prevent our body from eliminating as much as possible. If we obstruct our body's elimination functions, our body will not be able to thoroughly rid itself of waste matter, which is

True Beauty Story

MYA PALERMO, AGE THIRTY-TWO, CAME TO SEE ME AFTER SHE HAD BEEN TRYING to become a 100 percent raw vegan for one year. She simply did not feel well. Her skin looked patchy, she had acne outbreaks, and she was still at least twelve pounds heavier than her ideal weight. She still had intense cravings for cooked food, cheese, French fries and many of her favorite old treats, and she was tired a lot of the time. She could not understand why she did not look and feel better. After all, she reasoned, how could she be heavy and tired when she was eating all raw food?

Mya's perspective is a common one. Most people mistakenly believe that changing their diet is *all* it takes to maximize energy and look their best. While dietary changes are key, the other side of the equation is making sure we are eating the right foods at the right time, which helps our body cleanse out old waste. If we don't cleanse properly, our body will become overloaded with toxicity and we will *still* not feel great, even if we have good quality foods in our diet. Mya was regularly eating improper Beauty Food Pairings, and she was eating light and heavy foods in the wrong order. She was eating heavy breakfasts and lunches that included lots of nuts and dehydrated foods.

We started rebalancing Mya's diet with some easily digestible cooked food in the evenings and a great deal of Probiotic & Enzyme Salad (more on this on page 199), adding a daily probiotic and some gravity-method colonics. We also changed the order and the combination of the foods she was eating, and started her on fresh green drinks until noon. Mya started feeling great, and within three months fifteen pounds simply melted right off her. Her skin cleared up, and her cravings diminished! All she needed to become her most beautiful self was changing her food order and combinations to maximize energy and cleanse on an ongoing basis.

constantly accumulating. Toxicity will build, weight will pile on and be harder to take off, and our beauty will fade drastically.

The typical breakfast foods, such as plain granola or toast with butter, even when properly combined, are concentrated starch foods that stay in the stomach for at least a few hours. But most of us are not even eating properly combined breakfasts! For example, a breakfast of an egg white omelet with whole-wheat toast or a bagel with low-fat cream cheese is an improperly combined, beauty-busting meal and can stay in the stomach for hours and hours, sucking our precious Beauty Energy.

Here's the irony: w*e cannot get energy from food until nutrients from that food have been absorbed in the small intestine.* With all these typical breakfast foods, at least a few hours must pass before we even get energy at all out of them. During those first few hours, they are still being digested in our stomach! Instead of gaining energy you will be *using* energy to break down and digest them, and a lot of energy at that, since the most common breakfasts incorporate bad food combining. Heavy breakfasts are a major cause of the notorious mid-morning slump. We've all had *those* days when we check the time on our computer or on our cell phone every two minutes and wonder with dread how the heck we will be able to stay awake the whole day!

If we don't eat a heavy breakfast, we won't get bogged down with any heavy digesting processes. As a result, we will be more alert and have way more energy through our morning. We will also extend our body's cleansing time for more hours every day—more time to cleanse out the sludge! You'll also be far more likely to make better food choices for the rest of the day.

When you first start eating Light to Heavy, you may be used to eating heavier breakfast foods, and you may feel hungry at breakfast and want something that feels substantial. That is normal, because we have developed certain breakfast habits and our body is "used" to getting heavier at that time. As long as we put fibrous and water-containing veggies, like celery sticks or green drinks (discussed in the next chapter), in the body first, we can eat heavier foods afterward, like toast or whole-grain cereal with almond milk, while we are transitioning our system. There are more detailed steps on transitioning for breakfast in Part 2.

Over time we will feel so great from eating light earlier in the day that our cravings will greatly subside. *Trust me.* I used to really be a breakfast girl and would wake up starving in the morning and have big morning feasts. It was not unusual for me to have a banana, an orange, tea with almond milk, and a few pieces of sprouted bread or a big bowl of granola or, back in the day, two eggs. I was able to overcome that habit, the way we all can, over time. By sticking to light mornings, I feel infinitely better throughout my entire day. It is not an exaggeration to say that light mornings have improved my entire life! I am very grateful for the freed-up energy I enjoy from not having to obsess over my food choices—and I can *see* the differences it's made in my body and beauty, from my skin to my hair and nails, not to mention how easy it is to maintain my perfect weight!

Of course, some of us like to enjoy the occasional hearty brunch on vacation or on the weekend with friends or family. Don't worry. You won't have to ban brunch forever, as our bodies can deal with the occasional off-wagon event. What we want to focus on are everyday habits and patterns that we repeat over and over again.

Try it out for yourself! See how you feel shifting to lighter breakfasts for three weeks; then try to go back to the heavier way of eating breakfast. You won't want to, because you will feel *so* much better. You'll realize the heavy breakfasts really were making you tired. There is no stronger proof than personal experience.

LUNCH

We should eat lunch later on in our day, depending on when we get up in the morning. We eat lunch after we have set up our morning with a light breakfast, and when we start to feel truly hungry.

After breakfast, lunch is the most important meal to tackle, because we can extend cleansing and increase our Beauty Energy, or we can cause a traffic jam right in the middle of the day. When this happens, we slow everything down, so we can say goodbye to facilitating our weight-loss and beauty goals. For these reasons, we avoid eating concentrated protein at lunchtime, whether it's an animal source (chicken, fish, etc.) or a vegetarian one (nuts, seeds, etc.).

Proteins are the most difficult of all foods to digest, so we should save protein-based meals for the evening. The chances of causing a traffic jam go way up if we stick concentrated protein in the middle of the day. That would be that sixteen-wheel truck stuck right in the middle! And if we do not practice proper Beauty Food Pairing at lunch, forget about dinner! Even a superlight dinner would be sitting on top of food that is still digesting, as improper food combinations can take many hours to get through the stomach.

When we eat a dense, heavy lunch, we sacrifice our afternoons to sluggishness and low energy. We will get taken down like a rock before we ever saw it coming! Much of our body's energy will be directed to our belly to work to digest our heavy meal. Our mental abilities will deteriorate, and it will be a struggle to make it through the afternoon, let alone be motivated to go to the gym or a yoga class, or to spend an evening out with friends. This is usually when the second round of skinny lattes and Diet Cokes start to creep onto our desks and into our hands. Our bodies simply don't have enough energy during the day to digest major heavy foods *and* allow us to function at our peak.

Concerned about not getting enough protein in your diet if you cut out the concentrated protein from lunch? Remember our gorilla friends, who are the strongest and most muscular animals and eat greens for lunch and for pretty much every meal. We already discussed our true protein needs in Chapter 1, and we will also cover the topic of protein further in Chapter 5, Beauty Foods (page 83).

True Beauty Story

SANDY MONTAK, AGE FIFTY-ONE, IS A WARM, MOTHERLY CLIENT OF MINE WHO WORKS at an inner-city school with children that have learning disabilities. She was reluctant to change any of her food habits at first, but she knew she had to do something. She had high blood pressure, was obese and looked like she was at least in her sixties...a decade older than her real age. The first thing we focused on was her breakfast. Previously, she was eating three times before noon. She ate something as soon as she woke up "for energy," before she was even hungry, then ate a substantial breakfast mid-morning, followed by a fruit snack before lunchtime.

The first thing we did was replace all three mini prelunch meals with the Glowing Green Smoothie, followed by a small avocado or a piece of gluten-free toast if she was still hungry at least twenty minutes later. We did not change the rest of her day.

At first she was hungry and missed her heavy breakfasts enormously, but as she started to transition, she became much less hungry. She stuck to the morning routine, and after six weeks of keeping her mornings light, she had already lost twelve pounds. She started going to the bathroom a lot more, and her energy increased tenfold. We are still working toward improving lunch and the rest of her meals, but she is infinitely better off than she was when we first met—just by changing the first part of her day!

What about all that hype we hear that lunch should be heavier than dinner so we can "work off the calories"? Remember that we are not just looking at the caloric content of food. We are chiefly concerned with how efficiently and quickly our meals digest, and how little they contribute to sludge and use up our Beauty Energy, our real secret for burning off fat and keeping it off.

Two independent studies conducted in America and Germany used lab rats to display how eating *less* can often have positive effects. The experimental group was fed once a day for a two-hour period, while the control group was permitted to eat at will throughout the day. Both research teams found that the rats in the experimental group, which did not eat small amounts all day long, had higher enzyme activities in the fat cells and pancreas, and lower body weight. The American research team also found that the rats in the experimental group had a 17 percent longer lifespan.[22]

🍃 BEAUTY **TIP**

Grazing Accelerates Aging!

It is commonly believed we should eat small meals often to keep our metabolism up and stabilize blood sugar.

The truth, however, is that eating often is a sure way to age faster. There are different types of enzymes in our bodies that are involved with many different kinds of functions, including all digestive and metabolic processes, rebuilding the collagen in our skin, and maintaining our basic life force and vitality. Our diminishing enzyme pool is associated with the process of aging. Every time we eat, digestion has to be kicked back up, and so does the consumption of our body's precious enzymes. Constantly grazing throughout the day is a sure way to burn our body's enzymes more quickly...*and* speed up the aging process.

Grazing also ensures we are constantly packing more food on top of food that hasn't digested fully. The reality is most people end up eating *more* food when they graze. Grazing also slows the passage of food through our system. The slower foods move through, the greater the chance of creating fermented matter, putrefaction and gas—the toxicity that contributes to aging.

SLOW PASSAGE OF FOOD = FAST AGING

The foods we are going to eat throughout the day on the Beauty Detox are packed with natural dietary fiber, which helps control our blood sugar levels and keep them steady without having to nosh all day long.

DINNER

We've kept ourselves light and the path clear for proper digestion all the way until the evening. Excellent! Now we can enjoy a nice dinner with some heavier foods, depending on what our body needs and is calling for. Generally, we want to wait at least four hours after lunch to eat dinner, to give us enough time to properly digest the midday meal. We must be sure that we eat a lunch that satiates us for that period.

Excessive snacking between lunch and dinner can throw our digestive system into more turmoil and cause a traffic jam. It gives our digestive tract something new it suddenly has to deal with. Sure, it may perk up our metabolism temporarily, but it will also take more of our Beauty Energy and tax our digestive tract. However, the reality is that many of us are used to snacking and may want something to nosh on before dinner. If we do need a snack, the ideal snack would be something neutral, like vegetable sticks dipped in salsa or veggie dip, vegetable soup, or more of our lunch salad.

Dinner should always start with a green salad. Then, depending on our Beauty Detox phase and our motivation, it should be followed by a wide variety of foods. This is where animal protein fits into the Beauty Detox, if you choose to eat it. Why is this appropriate for dinner and not lunch? By dinnertime, our busy daytime activities and demands, both physical and mental, are now finished. We can relax and enjoy some social bonding time

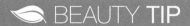

BEAUTY TIP

Eat Delicious Desserts That Won't Set You Back!

Have no fear! In moderation, we can still enjoy dessert on the Beauty Detox plan. What would life be without the occasional tasty treats, consumed for pure enjoyment?

Easily digestible desserts are important so we stay satisfied on the plan and don't feel deprived. The desserts we will be making are so delicious, you won't miss the bad-for-you stuff—the dairy, refined flour, refined sugar, processed soy, eggs, butter, trans fat, wheat, gluten, high fructose corn syrup, heated oils and artificial sweeteners—that make up most other popular desserts. *Those* are the ingredients that give desserts a bad name, and with good reason. They are toxic, clogging and aging.

Instead, we will be using ingredients such as stevia, moderate amounts of unrefined coconut oil and the occasional dark chocolate or raw cacao. We won't be cooking or baking at excessive temperatures, so, as you'll discover in Chapter 4, Beauty Minerals and Enzymes, the tasty desserts will retain their own enzymes so they will digest well and not set us back in our diet.

with our family and friends. We know we don't have to rush back to work. Because we have avoided a traffic jam during the entire day, thereby optimizing digestion and facilitating cleansing, we can now feel free to have some denser foods that we enjoy.

If we are going to veer off the plan (as we all will from time to time!) and improperly combine food groups, dinner would be the time to do it. Why? We've learned that improperly combined foods need hours to travel out of the stomach. Since we are improperly combining at the end of the day, we should allow that meal the time it needs to digest by not eating after it. If we have an improperly combined dinner at, say, 7:00 p.m., and we don't have breakfast until 10:00 a.m. the next morning, that is a full fifteen hours that we have allowed that food to move out of the stomach. On the other hand, if we *miscombine* at lunch, we've caused a traffic jam. Even if we eat fruit or a very light dinner later on in the day, those foods will sit on top of the poorly digesting lunchtime foods and will putrefy, ferment and spoil. There simply aren't enough hours in the day to eat a miscombined lunch! One of the easiest ways to compound toxicity is to eat more food of any kind after an ill-combined meal. Therefore, dinner should be our heavier meal, not lunch.

That said, we don't want to eat *right* before we go to bed. When possible, it is best to eat dinner at least three to four hours before bedtime, as food will pass through the digestive tract faster when we are awake. By eating this way, we will wake up feeling refreshed and energetic!

Your *New* Beauty Food Plan

BREAKFAST
New Belief: We won't eat until we are hungry. A lack of hunger means our bodies do not need food. When we do get hungry, we stick to light foods through the morning.

LUNCH
New Belief: Lunch is light and always properly combined so we can maintain optimal digestion and ongoing cleansing throughout the day.

DINNER
New Belief: Dinner is the time when we can relax a bit about our food choices, since we've eaten so well during the day and allowed our bodies to cleanse all day long. We aim to eat dinner three to four hours before we go to bed so that our food has time to digest optimally.

There is another reason that we incorporate heavier or cooked foods later in the day. It's important to transition our diets gradually, making sure we don't make a drastic switch to any kind of diet plan too quickly. By slowing the cleansing process at the end of the day with heavier or cooked foods at dinner, we avoid detoxing too much, too quickly, but we still make incredible progress, since we are staying clear and light during our *entire* day. The extra hours of ongoing cleansing really start to add up the more days we keep the path clear.

BEAUTY **DETOX** RECAP

- It is not just what we eat that counts, but what nutrients we are *able to use* from what we eat. When digestion is slow, a good deal of our food can ferment and putrefy, which creates unusable material for the body.

- When we practice proper Beauty Food Pairings, we will free up a lot of Beauty Energy from digestion, which can be used to rebuild our skin and hair, make us feel more energetic in our everyday lives and make weight loss easy.

- Photocopy the Beauty Food Pairing Cheat Sheet and consult it until you're familiar with how to optimally combine foods.

- Eat Light to Heavy throughout the whole day to free up Beauty Energy and promote sustained weight loss.

- Refer to Your New Beauty Food Plan to familiarize yourself with the basic framework of eating Light to Heavy throughout the day.

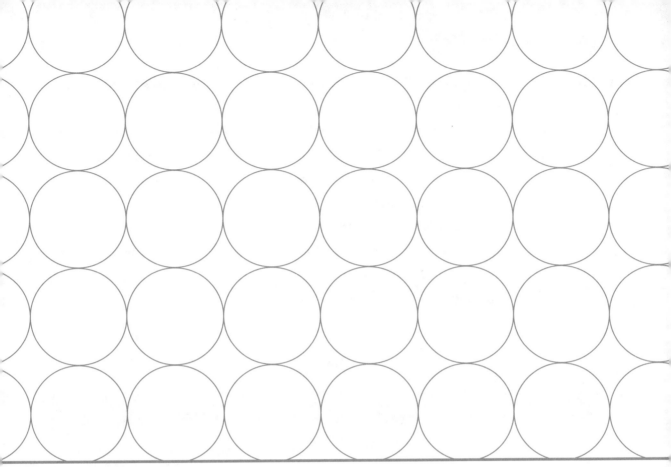

CHAPTER FOUR

BEAUTY MINERALS AND ENZYMES

Think of the fierce energy concentrated in an acorn! You bury it in the ground, and it explodes into a giant oak. Bury a sheep, and nothing happens but decay.

—George Bernard Shaw

Now that we've gone through the basic paradigm of our eating plan, let's talk about two key elements that contribute to beauty—minerals and enzymes.

Minerals are one of the keys to beauty, and an incredible 95 percent of our body's activities involve minerals. Our own body's biochemistry is dependent on our mineral sources. As you'll find out in this chapter, it is easy to provide the body with the essential minerals it needs when we are eating correctly.

Enzymes are the catalysts for hundreds of different processes in the body, including the rebuilding and renewal of skin collagen. Certain enzymes do not become truly active until the right quantities of trace and major minerals are present. And, we need living, active enzymes to fully absorb and assimilate our beauty minerals. Minerals and enzymes are best friends!

BEAUTY TIP

Get Your Dream Hair!

Our hair is part of our body, and our living hair follicles are rooted in our scalp, where they get their nutrition to be strong and healthy. I have personally experienced a dramatic transformation in my own hair since I started following the Beauty Detox Solution. In the past, my hair was a limp mess—I used to have to always pull it into a bun. Or I would have to allow up to an hour a day to blow-dry and style it to make it look presentable. But when I started the Beauty Detox, my hair became thick and bouncy. Now I just comb it in the shower and let it air-dry, and it looks good. Thank goodness it improved!

Thin, lifeless hair is an indication of a larger and more involved issue. We can't just focus on the hair specifically without taking the overall health of our body into account, just as with our skin. Though it is true that we all have different textures and hair types, when our hair is brittle or prematurely turning gray, it can be an indication that the body is lacking specific minerals and our diet must change to meet our body's needs. We can't just depend on expensive hair salon products! Until we work to alkalize and cleanse out some of our internal blockages, we cannot completely absorb the minerals present in our food or specific supplements.

You will find that the principles we apply to make our skin radiant and our weight effortlessly peel off our body are the same principles that will help bring that healthy sheen and bounce back to our hair. Increasing your intake of alkaline and mineral-rich foods, while simultaneously cleansing the clogging, acidic waste matter from your system, will increase your hair's vitality and give you those shampoo-commercial locks.

ESSENTIAL BEAUTY MINERALS

Where do minerals come from? They primarily come from the soil, which is why the quality of soil is so important, and why we want to buy as much organic produce as possible, since organic soil has a higher mineral content than traditional farming soil. Some studies show up to 87 percent more minerals in certain organic fruits and vegetables![1] The minerals filter into plants through the water in the soil, which contains the wide spectrum of soluble minerals that are absorbed into plants, then move through the plants' stems, and out into their leaves. Eating plants is like eating pure sun energy and pure mineral content.

Green plants are our number one food group for providing us with all the minerals that we need for superior beauty and nutrition, while simultaneously giving us the vitamins and the amino acids that we need to build protein. If we eat greens abundantly and get a good variety of them in our diet, we will inherently get the wide spectrum of minerals we need into our bodies. Greens are also among our strongest detox weapons, since their powerful alkalinity helps root poison out the more consistently we consume them!

The High-Mineral Foods chart is a *partial* list of high mineral-containing greens and other foods. Animal proteins, which we learned are complex to digest and leave acidic residue in our bodies, are allowed in moderation for those that really want to keep them in the diet, but are not included below since we do not rely on them for the majority of our minerals.

ENZYMES BUILD BEAUTY

In the mainstream health world we often hear about measuring a food's worth by its protein, calorie and carbohydrate content. But what about enzymes? As you will discover, in the words of natural health pioneer Dr. Ann Wigmore, "enzyme preservation is the secret to health." Dr. Wigmore isn't the only researcher to underscore the importance of enzymes. Dr. Troland of Harvard University once said, "Life is something which has been built up about the enzyme; it is a corollary of enzyme activity." And to that quote, I'd like to add that enzymes are also a major secret to beauty!

Live enzymes are the catalyst for every human function. They are, as Dr. Edward Howell, one of the fathers of food enzyme research, said, "chemical protein complexes and bioenergy reservoirs." Scientists have identified over five thousand different enzymes that

High-Mineral Foods

HIGH MINERAL-CONTAINING GREENS		
Arugula	Cucumber	Radicchio
Bok choy	Dandelion	Romaine lettuce (and green and red leaf)
Broccoli	Escarole	Spinach
Celery	Frisée	Swiss chard
Chard	Kale (three types)	Watercress
Collard greens	Mustard greens	Wheatgrass

HIGH MINERAL-CONTAINING HERBS		
Basil	Dill	Mint
Cilantro	Fennel	Parsley (two types)

HIGH MINERAL-CONTAINING VEGETABLES		
Asparagus	Endive	Radishes
Beets	Green beans	Rutabaga
Bell peppers	Jerusalem artichokes	Sea vegetables, all types
Broccoli	Leek	Squash, all varieties
Brussels sprouts	Mushrooms	Sweet potatoes
Cabbage	Okra	Tomatoes
Carrots	Onions	Turnips
Cauliflower	Parsnip	Yams
Eggplant	Peas	Zucchini

High-Mineral Foods

HIGH MINERAL-CONTAINING SPROUTS		
Alfalfa	Clover	Sunflower
Broccoli	Radish	

HIGH MINERAL-CONTAINING FRUITS		
Acai berries	Durian	Oranges
Apples	Figs	Papaya
Avocado	Goji berries	Pears
Bananas	Grapefruit	Pineapples
Blackberries	Grapes	Plums
Blueberries	Huckleberries	Pomegranate
Cherimoya	Lemons	Strawberries
Cherries	Limes	Tangerines
Cucumbers	Olives	

HIGH MINERAL-CONTAINING NUTS AND SEEDS		
Almonds	Hemp seeds	Pumpkin seeds
Brazil nuts	Macadamia nuts	Sesame seeds
Cacao	Pecans	Sunflower seeds
Coconuts	Pine nuts	Walnuts

HIGH MINERAL-CONTAINING ROOTS		
Ginger	Maca	Turmeric

our bodies utilize and manufacture, but there may be far more.[2] Enzymes are catalysts of biochemical reactions in living beings and perform thousands of important life-supporting functions. For example, enzymes help repair our DNA, help digest our food and help us assimilate the nutrients within food. They repair and prevent wrinkles, help even our skin tone and contribute to smooth, youthful skin. Enzymes also help speed up weight loss and detoxification as they free up more metabolic energy. We need as many enzymes as possible to support these functions.

We were born with a huge enzyme reserve, but this reserve decreases over time, causing aging and a slowing of the metabolism. Dr. Meyer and his research associates at Michael Reese Hospital in Chicago found that the enzyme level in adults aged twenty-one to thirty-one was thirty times greater than in adults aged sixty-nine to one hundred.

🍃 BEAUTY TIP

A Few of the Top Beauty Minerals

SILICON: Makes our hair thick, our nails strong, and increases our vitality. It is also excellent for smooth, beautiful skin and can improve wrinkles. Silicon also strengthens the connective tissues and bones and helps keep us flexible.

ZINC: Helps rebuild our collagen to make the skin healthy, glowing and smooth, and helps prevent wrinkles, stretch marks, radiation damage and other signs of aging.

IRON: Generates a magnetic blood current, as iron is the center of the hemoglobin molecule, which carries oxygen throughout the body. Healthy, oxygenated blood stimulates healthy circulation, resulting in a gorgeous, highly attractive glow in the skin. Iron also boosts our energy levels and immunity, while encouraging restful sleep.

MAGNESIUM: Opens up three hundred different detoxification pathways in the body and is a key mineral for keeping our bowels regular, a crucial part of our ongoing cleansing program. A strengthening beauty mineral, magnesium helps the bones absorb calcium and plays an important role in converting vitamin D to its active hormonal form.

POTASSIUM: Is an essential balancing mineral. Since potassium is an electrolyte, we rely on it to maintain our body's proper fluid levels. It helps balance the levels of other minerals, especially sodium. Potassium is needed for cellular cleansing, as it regulates the transfer of nutrients into cells and is crucial for the elimination of wastes.

CALCIUM: Is a strengthening mineral, as it helps keep our bones strong, our posture upright, and enables us to move gracefully.

True Beauty Story

PAT DAVIS IS A CLIENT OF MINE WHO IS THIRTY-NINE YEARS OLD AND HAS three children under the age of twelve. She spends the majority of her time running after her children, including the youngest, who is two years old. When she drove into the city from New Jersey to meet me for the first time, she was thin and pale—almost fragile looking—with a dusting of freckles. Her light brown hair was incredibly thin and full of split ends. But what I noticed most of all was her skin. It was uneven and dull, she had dark circles under her eyes and her face looked droopy. My first thought was that this woman was way too young to be aging this quickly!

Overeating and losing weight were not the issues; restoring her beauty was. I could tell that she was eating a diet deficient in alkaline minerals, and her skin publicly announced that to the entire world. No amount of makeup could make up for the lack of radiant skin and a healthy, toxin-free blood flow to her face. She had spent over a decade focusing on the health and well-being of her children, and now she was ready to start focusing on herself and liking how she looked again.

Her diet turned out be very rich in highly refined starches and had hardly any greens or other vegetables. It was made up of Cheerios, bagels, tuna fish or ham sandwiches on rye bread, Pop-Tarts, and pretty much whatever her kids liked eating. For dinner she made a lot of chicken and rice dishes, mac and cheese, rice and beans, or any other combo that was easy to make for her large family.

We started exploring ways she could bring in more Beauty Minerals, such as by consuming a much larger amount of greens and other vegetables. She started having the Glowing Green Smoothie every morning, making it in batches to last two days, so she could save time by making it only every other day. I showed her how to make easy, tasty green salads that she could toss together while making her kids' lunches and dinners, so she wouldn't feel like she was making two completely different meals. We also incorporated some cleansing aids, including eating lots of Probiotic & Enzyme Salad, and taking a daily probiotic supplement and digestive enzymes. We always have to address not only adding *in* healthy new foods but also working on cleaning *out* the old sludge.

After a few weeks her skin already looked more smooth and plumped up, and many of the fine lines on her face had diminished. Her eyes shone with an inner light, and the cracked edges of her lips had healed and her lips had started to plump up. Now it has been over eight months since we started working together. Her hair has developed a gorgeous sheen, and her face literally looks ten years younger. While she is actually making different foods for herself and her kids for many of their meals, she still feels like she has *more* energy and *more* time on her hands. She is now one very sexy mom! I look forward to being a witness to her growing younger and younger as the years go on.

Our goal with the Beauty Detox Solution is to preserve as many of our enzymes as possible. Think about it: if we have *fewer* enzymes working for us, their priority has to be the major processes that help us to stay alive, like digestion and blood rebuilding. This fits right in with Beauty Energy. Enzymes are essential for our vitality and increase our Beauty Energy. What if we had a *plentiful* supply of enzymes in our system? You guessed it! The enzymes would be able to tend to both the major processes and those lower on the body's totem pole of priorities (but that are very important to us), like tending to our limp hair and the crow's-feet around our eyes!

One way to do this is to infuse our body with enzymes, which are found in raw plant foods. The more of this living fuel we eat, the more alive we will feel! Enzymes are heat-sensitive entities. Though they hold up pretty well in the freezer, they become denatured and damaged at about 118 degrees F, and die at temperatures just above that. This makes sense if you think about the fact that fire does not add; it takes away. Have you ever burned your finger with a match or by picking up something really hot? The skin on your finger turned red and then possibly even black, as the cells were destroyed.

It is the same process with vegetables. Take a look at a head of vibrant green kale. It is so incredibly thick and waxy that when you go to wash it, the water molecules slip right off it, just like they do on the mighty leafy plants in the Amazon jungle, which could shade us from a torrential downpour. Now sauté that kale, fry it in a heated pan, and watch how the very vibrancy of the leaves fades. The leaves acquire a soft, mushy consistency and absorb water. Their powerful energy has been broken down.

When we cook our food, we kill off the enzymes and diminish the vibrancy of the food itself. When we constantly eat food with diminished vibrancy, our own "oomph" factor starts to fizzle. We directly take in the energy of the food that we con-

Why You've Never Seen an Old Wild Animal

Unless a wild animal is *really* old or sick and close to death, have you ever noticed that you can't really tell how old it is? I noticed this throughout the eleven African safaris I went on during my world journey, in such countries as Zimbabwe, Zambia, Botswana, Tanzania and Swaziland.

Domesticated animals and pets start to look old and weathered over time. They also get degenerative diseases like we do, such as arthritis, cancer and type 2 diabetes! Well, it makes sense, because unlike wild animals, they are usually fed processed and pre-packaged food!

sume. Therefore, to promote our rejuvenation process, we need to load up on our living food friends: the mighty enzymes. Life begets life.

Enzyme-rich foods are also uniquely designed to help us digest them, and this helps us lose weight. How? The enzymes in raw foods alleviate some of the work that our digestive enzymes have to do to break down and digest food. The three basic digestive enzymes we're concerned with are amylases, proteases and lipases, which are the specific digestive enzymes used to break down starches, proteins and fats, respectively. Let's use the example of fats to demonstrate what happens when we cook our food. When you eat avocados, for instance, the lipase in the avocado helps you digest the avocado without taxing your digestive enzyme reserves. But let's say you're going to use olive oil to cook a vegetable. The fat in the olive oil gets heated to high temperatures, killing off its lipase enzymes. Without the lipase in the olive oil, you need to use more of your lipase enzymes to digest the fat. Not only do you use more digestive enzymes, but you run the risk of that olive oil contributing to the sludge (and ultimately to your body fat) since it doesn't digest as easily.

Again, this is not the case with a raw plant fat, such as an avocado, which will digest in the stomach with its own lipase enzymes. This is why raw nuts are much less fattening than roasted nuts!

Wait, you might be thinking, *there-are centuries-old culinary traditions that rely on heating and processing foods.... And don't we have enough enzymes to digest our food?* Sure we do, but that doesn't mean we need to overly rely on them. Doing so takes enzymes away from the myriad of other things they can do for your body. The Beauty Detox is all about *maximizing*

Beauty Detox Digestive Enzymes

SPECIFIC ENZYME	BREAKS DOWN...
Amylase	Starch
Protease	Protein
Lipase	Fat

your body's potential, and part of that is preserving—and even increasing— your enzyme reserves.

This is not to suggest that we must eat 100 percent raw foods. Easily digestible cooked food has its place also. But it does mean that we need to increase the percentage of raw greens and vegetables we consume overall. As you learned in Chapter 3, it is important to always consume raw plant foods at the beginning of every meal. That could mean a salad or simply a few celery sticks. We can build sensibly from there, but starting each meal with these raw greens and other veggies will ensure that we are increasing our enzyme intake. This alone will start rebuilding our beauty and adding to our Beauty Energy. And enzymes aren't the only heat-sensitive entities on our list. Vitamins and other nutrients also respond to temperature. When we eat *all* cooked food, our organs do not get as many nutrients as they do when we consume raw food, and we tend to eat more to feel satiated.

True Beauty Story

JULIAN DE VITO IS A THIRTY-EIGHT-YEAR-OLD MAN WITH A VERY BUSY PRODUCTION and publicity career in Hollywood. When he was working on a movie, it was not unusual for him to gain twenty pounds over the course of three months, due to stress and the ubiquitous snack service stations stocked with junk food. Overall, he was about forty pounds overweight. At his young age, he already had high blood pressure and, thanks in part to his raging sweet tooth, he was an ideal diabetes candidate.

He periodically undertook a weight loss program in which he would eat only the prepackaged, microwaved food products that this particular diet program required. He would go on the program for a few weeks at a time, drop a bunch of weight, then gain it back a few weeks later. I don't know what was more horrifying: his yo-yo weight loss efforts and the strain they put on his poor body, or the amount of processed, preservative-filled, "dead" food he ate regularly on these weight loss programs, which only created more sludge in his body.

We started working together, and I put him on a transition diet with an emphasis on eating unprocessed foods with their natural enzymes intact through the first part of his day. He always started his meal with a raw salad or vegetable, and increased the overall percentage of unprocessed food in his diet. He cut out acidic or processed foods, such as grilled chicken sandwiches and commercial cereal with skim milk.

He loved the easy recipes I taught him, and realized that it was simple to make salads and other dishes taste amazing, and that there were so many great options. In eight months he shed his forty-two extra pounds and got the added bonus of glowing skin. People even started telling him he looked like he was in his late twenties (not a bad thing when you work in Hollywood)! It has been over two years now since Julian and I started working together, and he has broken the cycle of yo-yoing and kept the weight off. He currently weighs in at 160 pounds, down from the 205 pounds he weighed when I met him—an ideal weight for his five-foot-nine-inch frame.

By starting our meals with raw greens and other raw vegetables, we load up on some enzymes right at the start to help us digest the rest of our food. We also feel fuller faster since these foods contain so much fiber, and we can eat them in abundance while still eating fewer overall calories.

WHERE COOKED FOOD FITS IN

Even while the majority of what you eat should be enzyme-rich raw food, there is definitely room for the right kind of cooked food in your diet. In fact, cooked food plays a beneficial role, as it brings some heaviness and grounding to the diet. We always start our meals with some raw vegetables or greens, but we can follow with some high-quality cooked food, especially at dinner. For people with weak digestive systems, lightly cooked vegetables, such as broccoli, may digest better than raw ones. Starchy vegetables, such as sweet potatoes and yams, digest better when they are very well cooked. And high-quality, gluten-free cooked grains, such as quinoa, are excellent for us to include in our diet.

MINERALS + ENZYMES = GREEN DRINKS

The absolute most powerful way to simultaneously up our mineral and enzyme consumption is to consume green drinks every day, specifically the Glowing Green Smoothie (see page 197) and the Glowing Green Juice (see page 198). In green drinks we condense the vegetables and fruits by blending or juicing and, in so doing, multiply the quantities of enzymes and minerals we obtain. Green-based drinks are the *real* super foods—not exotic, expensive or hard-to-find fruits or plants from foreign countries.

Perhaps you are thinking, *How many days a week do I have to do that?* or *For how long do I have to that?* And my counterquestion back to you is, "How many days do you want to be healthy and beautiful?" Remember this is not a quick-fix answer to detoxify and look great but a way to permanently break out of our old habits. To maximize our intake of minerals and enzymes, we should aim to consume the Glowing Green Smoothie or the Glowing Green Juice *every* day.

But don't fret. The green drinks are delicious! The fruit cuts right through any "green" taste and makes for a balanced, enjoyable flavor. You will be pleasantly surprised with your first sip! When I drink them, I get a rush of sustained energy that lasts for hours, I feel clearheaded, calm, and it is much easier to focus on work or any tasks at hand. I can't wait for you to experience the same thing! The great news is that as the biochemistry of your body changes and your looks and energy start to improve, you will actually look forward to your green drinks. Seriously! I have had tons of clients report back months later that they are now addicted to their morning ritual.

Think having a blended vegetable drink sounds weird? Don't want to invest in a blender at this time? You are not alone and it is totally okay. In the Blossoming Beauty phase you will not have to make or consume these green drinks. The Blossoming Beauty phase still provides for powerful cleansing and improvement by incorporating all the other principles we talked about. Down the road, as you start to experience great results and your body becomes cleaner, you may be interested in going further and revisiting the green drinks, which come into play beginning in the Radiant Beauty phase.

True Beauty Story

AARON STEINER IS A FORTY-SOMETHING-YEAR-OLD BANKER. SINCE HE DEALS WITH trading stock, he usually gets to his office by 5:30 a.m. When I met him, he was consuming five cups of coffee *before* noon, and he was still in a perpetual energy slump. After work he ate some kind of quick dinner, then usually passed out right away. He never felt good or felt that he had any real energy to do anything. He was literally dragging himself through life—if you can call that living!

He did not want to change his lunches and dinners very much, since they were often either rushed or at fancy restaurants with clients. But the one thing he did agree to have every morning was a Glowing Green Smoothie on his way to work. I brought his wife on board and she started making them for the both of them. Within a week Aaron reported to me that he was feeling much more energetic and was already cutting back on coffee. Within six weeks he was down to one and a half cups of coffee for the whole day and was dropping weight. At the four-month mark he was still drinking one and a half cups of coffee, but he had lost fifteen pounds, his cholesterol numbers had improved considerably and he had more energy than he had had in years! He had even started to practice yoga on the weekends and one night during the week. While he cut back on his meat intake and made some other improvements, it was the Glowing Green Smoothie that really made the major difference.

Over time, as your body's makeup shifts, you will start rooting out the blockages and poisons that are causing cravings for the heavier foods or caffeinated beverages that you consumed in the past. And you will start loving how the green drinks make you feel light and energetic and, yes, how they improve your appearance and help you drop the pounds!

GLOWING GREEN SMOOTHIE

I've been talking about my Glowing Green Smoothie on my website and in the press for years. It is based on Dr. Ann Wigmore's philosophy of blended food, which I learned about firsthand at her institute in Puerto Rico. Dr. Wigmore studied cellular nutritional healing for over thirty-five years. One of her major theories is that by blending foods before eating them, you "predigest" them, so the body does not have to work to break down the foods and waste unnecessary energy in digestion. *Remember our Beauty Energy principle?*

Many of the important minerals and other nutrients in food are encased in the cell walls, and these need to be ruptured to extract the nutrients. Thus, blending helps make the greens' full spectrum of nutrition readily available to the body without the body doing any work. We also add some fresh fruit, which really balances the taste of the greens. Served cold, the Glowing Green Smoothie is delicious!

What is so wonderful about the Glowing Green Smoothie is that you retain the

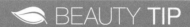
BEAUTY TIP
Nix the Caffeine

When we ingest caffeine, it is absorbed throughout the body and affects many of our critical organs, interfering with numerous processes in the body. Caffeine is particularly taxing on the liver, which has to metabolize it. Too much caffeine can overload the liver and slow down the liver's ability to efficiently burn fat and cleanse out other toxins in our system. Caffeine can also contribute to increased levels of cortisol, a stress hormone that has been linked to excess fat storage, especially around our bellies. Caffeine can also promote norepinephrine production, which is another stress hormone that affects our brain and nervous system, raising our heart rate and blood pressure. It creates that jittery feeling we may be familiar with after having even just one or two cups of coffee!

This is one of the reasons I don't recommend drinking much green tea, and why I personally avoid it. Even though green tea contains some healthy antioxidants, one cup has around thirty-five milligrams of caffeine. White tea, with only about eight milligrams of caffeine per cup, or better yet, caffeine-free rooibos tea and herbal teas are much better choices, and they contain antioxidants, such as aspalathin and nothofagin.

integrity of the whole vegetables and fruits, so you still enjoy all the fiber. When we move into this new way of eating, fiber is one of our best friends, as it helps to sweep up the newly awakened poisons and helps strengthen our bowel movements. The high volume of fiber in the Glowing Green Smoothie keeps us feeling full throughout the morning and up to lunch, especially in the beginning, when we are used to being stimulated by denser and heavier volumes of food.

GLOWING GREEN JUICE

If Dr. Ann Wigmore is the "mother" of the Glowing Green Smoothie, then I would consider the modern-day father of the Glowing Green Juice to be the delightful Dr. Norman Walker, who lived to be well over one hundred. The Glowing Green Juice is loaded with enzymes, oxygen, minerals and vitamins that, according to Dr. Walker, have been "liberated" from the other food components and are thus much easier to absorb into the intestinal wall. And because much of the good stuff is in the juice of plants, with a Glowing Green Juice you can take in even more of these nutrients, as well as the purest organic water on earth.

The Glowing Green Juice is pure liquid nutrition that will fuel our bodies. As we cleanse and become more alkaline, we need less stimulation from solid food in the morning, and the Glowing Green Juice provides enzymes, minerals and vitamins for our bodies and does not slow us down one bit. Since the Glowing Green Juice is stripped of fiber, it hits the system in a stronger cleansing way. For those that have a highly acidic and toxic body, initially the Glowing Green Juice can be too much of a shock to consume every day. Until we start to shift the body into a more alkaline state, the more concentrated sugar content of the juiced fruit in the Glowing Green Juice can also be too much for the system, as fruits are the strongest cleansers. Since it lacks fiber, I have noticed with many of my clients that initially, the Glowing Green Juice may not keep them full enough for long periods the way the Glowing Green Smoothie does.

If we continue to have problems with fruit, even after adequate transition times, we can substitute stevia for the fruit in the Glowing Green Juice. The Glowing Green Juice comes into play in the True Beauty phase, *after* we have made some other necessary adjustments. In True Beauty we will consume both the Glowing Green Smoothie and the Glowing Green Juice depending on the rest of that day's meal plan. Many will skip the Glowing Green Juice and will stick with the Glowing Green Smoothie for even longer, or permanently, as they personally prefer it. I have many clients who have been on my plan for several years and, although they have the Glowing Green Juice occasionally and understand the theory of it, they prefer to stick with the fiber-containing Glowing Green Smoothie and function better with it. I personally regularly consume both.

You might be wondering about the juices available in stores. V8 and all the other pre-packaged, pre-bottled drinks simply don't count. The nature of the bottling process means that the juices have been pasteurized, and that means the vegetables and fruits have been heated to such high temperatures that the enzymes and much of the nutrition have been killed and denatured. It is literally the difference between life and death: choosing living green drinks made from living foods or heated, dead, enzyme-deficient drinks.

If it is easier for you from a time standpoint to make larger batches of green drinks and freeze them in portions, that is perfectly fine. So many of my clients do this. While fresh is ideal, enzymes and other nutrients hold up pretty well in the freezer. Don't worry about losing out on too much by freezing larger batches; you will still get plenty of minerals and nutrients from the drinks. It is more important that you stick to the plan and consume your green drinks every morning, rather than worry that you could not make the green drinks fresh some days.

True Beauty Story

MARY STEWART IS A THIRTY-NINE-YEAR-OLD WOMAN WHO HAD BEEN TRYING TO have a baby for thirteen years with her husband. They tried everything from in vitro fertilization to acupuncture. When I met them, they had already given up on the idea of conceiving their own child and had started looking into adoption options in the United States and other countries. It was around then that Mary called on me simply to improve her overall diet.

As we started working to make changes to her diet, she vacillated on sticking to her ideal lunch and dinner options, but she stayed true to one thing: her morning Glowing Green Smoothie. Within seven months of consuming it once or twice every single day, she became pregnant! The high quantity of greens, packed with minerals and chlorophyll, helped rebalance her body and made it healthy enough for her to carry a baby. Today she is the proud mother of a healthy nine-month-old son. She even named him after the street I live on!

Recipes for both the Glowing Green Smoothie and the Glowing Green Juice can be found in Chapter 11, Beauty Recipes (page 193). Remember that the recipes for the Glowing Green Smoothie and Glowing Green Juice I provide are mere guidelines. I get so many people emailing me to say, "I don't like celery. Can I switch to cucumber?" or "Ugh, please don't make me eat cilantro!" I won't! You can and should feel free to mix and match your greens and fruits, depending on what is local and seasonal and on your personal preferences. Think of your favorite fruits as your favorite go-to jeans, and your leafy greens as your many different cute tops. The jeans (or fruits, in this case) are really the support for the fabulous, eye-catching tops (or leafy greens), which are the most important part of the outfit.

True Beauty Story

MARGARET REILLY IS A TELEVISION PRODUCER IN HER EARLY THIRTIES—INCREDIBLY young to have the amount of responsibility she has been given. She works extremely hard and is also very stressed on a daily basis. When I met her, she needed to lose about twenty pounds. She was actually five days into the Master Cleanse, a liquid cleanse program, and while she had no energy, she was pleased that she had already lost four pounds. Still, she knew that she could not continue that drastic a cleanse while working as hard as she did, and she was looking for more of a long-term approach. In general, she ate lunch at her desk and ordered takeout for dinner. She had no energy to go to the gym or exercise in any way. She admitted that her lunches and dinners were her "treats," the parts of the day when she just got to eat what she wanted and temporarily feel good.

That left us with the perfect starting place: breakfast. I started her on the Glowing Green Smoothie every single day. At first she was still hungry afterward and ate some eggs "for protein"—her usual breakfast—but as we shifted, she found she needed only the Glowing Green Smoothie. Naturally, she started cutting back on her coffee and her lunches got lighter. After three months, she had lost a total of seventeen pounds. She had so much energy from her Glowing Green Smoothie that she started going to the gym at least three times a week.

Now it has been a year since I met Margaret. We have shifted other parts of her diet, and she has switched to the Glowing Green Juice, which is her only food until lunch. Then she always has a Glowing Green Smoothie as her afternoon snack. She has lost a total of twenty-five pounds, and she looks absolutely beautiful. Her face even looks different, as her jawline is more defined, and she has smoother, firmer skin. Her job is still stressful, but *she* does not get as stressed anymore. She is more grounded and much happier.

Variety will ensure you get a wide range of the key minerals, as different minerals are present in higher quantities in different greens. As you continue on this plan, you'll be surprised to see that your personal tastes and preferences for different greens will expand as we start to alter the biochemical makeup of your body. I used to not like kale that much, and avoided arugula at all costs, but now they are two of my staple faves. Who would have thought that would happen? So remember, as your body changes physically, so do your tastes. Also, choose seasonal and organic greens and fruits whenever possible! They don't have to travel very far to reach us, thus reducing our carbon footprint. They will also be more rich in minerals as they have more time to ripen in the field or orchard.

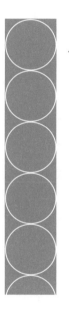

BEAUTY **DETOX** RECAP

○ Minerals are necessary to build our beauty. Our most plentiful sources of minerals are greens and other vegetables.

○ Enzymes help reverse the aging process, increase beauty and help us lose weight.

○ We start each meal with raw vegetables or greens to ensure we are getting a plentiful supply of enzyme-rich foods to increase our enzyme reserve.

○ Starting in the Radiant Beauty phase, the Glowing Green Smoothie and the Glowing Green Juice are an important part of the daily diet, providing us with large quantities of easily assimilated minerals and enzymes.

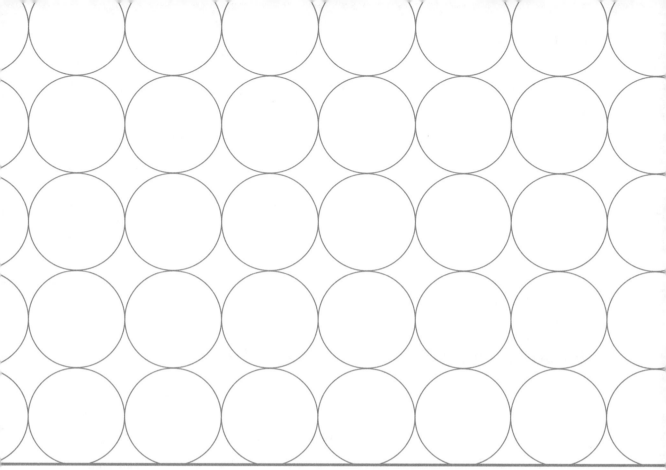

CHAPTER FIVE

BEAUTY FOODS

When we learn to eat properly, we begin to rebuild our bodies and to fulfill our purpose on this planet: to grow in health, creativity, wisdom and compassion.

—Dr. Ann Wigmore
Living Foods Lifestyle™ Textbook

Now that you understand the Beauty Detox concepts, it's time to get to the heart of the program: the food itself. This chapter introduces you to the variety of mineral- and enzyme-rich foods that will help you boost your Beauty Energy, cleanse the toxic sludge and reach new levels of beauty! I'll walk you through all the different foods we talked about earlier, with helpful tips along the way for how to incorporate them into your Beauty Detox.

To understand the foods that boost beauty, we're going to revisit the traditional nutrition categories. Remember to open your mind and forget all the mainstream nutrition talk you've heard over and over again. You know now that it isn't working! This chapter will introduce you to a new way to think about food and how your body uses it so that you can eat your way to a more beautiful you.

PLANT PROTEIN IS BEAUTY PROTEIN

Protein is a macronutrient composed of building blocks called amino acids, which link together to form protein chains in different combinations. Proteins perform many different functions in our body. To name a few, they maintain and foster the growth of our cells, make antibodies and hormones, and help regulate our fluid and electrolyte balance.

Protein is probably the most poorly understood category of foods there is. And no wonder! An ever-growing number of confusing studies and statistics are put out about protein. And while we have traded cutting out carb grams and fat grams during different dieting fads over the last few decades, it has never been suggested that we cut back on the highly touted, "royalty" macronutrient called protein. In fact, we are often led to believe that we can never consume too much protein! *Protein helps us lose weight, gives us muscle and skin tone . . . so cut back on calories, carbs, fat grams, yes, but never protein!* Does this sound familiar?

One of the first things that a vegetarian is asked is, "Where do you get your protein?" This highlights the misconception in our society that *only* meat and animal products contain protein, and if we do not eat it, we are at risk for protein deficiency. I admit that I used to wonder if I was getting enough protein when I stopped eating animal products altogether. I used to supplement my diet with protein powders and was sure to eat a certain amount of nuts a day. But I stopped these practices years ago, as I now know that I get more than enough protein from my plant-based diet, without trying to supplement protein. I feel better than ever, and my body is more toned than it has ever been!

Let's back up for a minute to get a wider view of this protein issue: *Our bodies do not use protein per se. It uses amino acids.* Long chains of amino acids make up proteins. These chains wear out and do need to be replaced. We furnish replacements for these proteins by consuming foods with *amino acid* building blocks.

Dr. T. Colin Campbell uses the great example of strings of multicolored beads in his book *The China Study* to explain how our bodies use amino acids. Say we lose a string of colored beads, and someone gives us another string of colored beads to replace it, but the beads are in a different order in terms of their color. In order to be able to use the new beads, we have to cut apart the whole string, then restring the beads in the right order.[1]

This is the basic concept we have to understand with protein: the amino acid chains need to be broken down so we can reconstruct their order in a specific way for our bodies. Our bodies cannot use a complex amino acid chain without rebuilding it first. Make sense? So while all organisms and plants have the same basic amino acids, the usable pattern is specific to each organism. We don't just eat chicken or beef and instantly absorb "protein" into our bodies. Instead, our body has to break down the amino acids from the chicken or beef that we ate, and then restring the amino acids into protein chains specific to humans.

Animal protein is defined as beef, chicken and all other fowl, venison, lamb, pork, rabbit, fish and other seafood, eggs and so on. We cannot just eat animal protein, which is really the muscle of the animal, and expect that to turn directly into muscle in our bodies. If that were the case, how does the cow itself, the source of big protein steaks and burgers, build muscle when it naturally eats only grass? The cow builds its large muscles from the *amino acids* in the grass it is eating!

Remember from our first discussion about the animal kingdom that many of the largest, most muscular animals on earth are vegetarians—gorillas, wild horses, hippos, rhinos. They efficiently build up the protein and muscles in their body from the amino acids in the greens they eat. The false idea of having to eat exclusively protein-dense food, namely animal protein, to build muscle has been popularized by mainstream nutrition and the media.

We have established that before muscle or tissue can be built up in the body, protein has to be digested and split into amino acids. There are twenty-three different amino acids, fifteen that the body manufactures on its own and eight that cannot be manufactured by the body and must come from our diet alone. When a food contains all eight of these amino acids—known as the essential amino acids—it is called a complete protein. These eight essential

The Essential Eight

The essential eight amino acids cannot be manufactured by the body, so we need to get these key protein-building blocks from the foods we eat.

phenylalanine	valine	lysine	leucine
isoleucine	tryptophan	threonine	methionine

amino acids are found in abundance in fruits, vegetables, seeds, sprouts and nuts. Some examples of great plant-based food sources of amino acids are all nuts and seeds, spinach, kale, broccoli, Brussels sprouts, cabbage, cauliflower, summer squash and asparagus.

By consuming a wide variety of foods from these various plant groups, you will receive the essential eight amino acids in abundance. Furthermore, you do not need to carefully combine foods to get all eight essential amino acids at each meal. A best-selling book in the 1960s called *Diet for a Small Planet* popularized the idea of "protein combining." But in 1981 the author herself, Frances Moore Lappé, rewrote the book to reflect that her previous theories of protein combining had been misinformed. Our bodies store and release the amino acids needed over a twenty-four-hour period to supplement our daily amino acid intake and ensure we get all the amino acids we need.[2]

DANGERS OF HIGH-PROTEIN DIETS

Over the past decade or so, a number of high-protein, low-carb diets have become increasingly popular. What you've read so far in this book points to exactly why these types of diets age us at an accelerated rate. These diets are based on extreme calorie restriction and focus on foods that lack fiber and nutrients. There are many potential health risks associated with these diets, as well.

A study published in 2002[3] and funded by the Atkins Center for Complementary Medicine researched fifty-one obese people that were put on the low-carb Atkins Diet.[4] Over six months forty-one subjects maintained the diet and lost an average of twenty pounds. Sound good? The participants in the study were consuming an average of only 1,450 calories per day, which is 35 percent less than the average American consumption of 2,250 calories a day.[5] On any kind of diet, if anyone were to restrict daily calories by at least 35 percent, he or she would lose weight, at least for the short term.

In the same study the researchers also stated that "at some point during the twenty-four weeks, twenty-eight subjects (68%) reported constipation, twenty-six (63%) reported bad breath, twenty-one (51%) reported headache, four (10%) noted hair loss, and one woman (1%) reported increased menstrual bleeding." Another frightening figure from the study is that dieters had a 53 percent increase in the amount of calcium excreted in their urine, which is a big problem for bone density and health.

One study published in the *Asia Pacific Journal of Clinical Nutrition* focusing on the short- and long-term effects of high-protein and low-carb diets found that "complications such as heart arrhythmias, cardiac contractile function impairment, sudden death, osteoporosis, kidney damage, increased cancer risk, impairment of physical activity and lipid abnormalities can all be linked to long-term restriction of carbohydrates in the diet."[6]

So don't be tempted by the low-carb diet craze—diets high in animal protein are simply *not* going to promote our beauty and health.

Since our body uses amino acids to construct the protein it needs, it is vital that we look not only at how many grams of protein we are eating but also at the *quality* of our foods' amino acids and how readily available they are. Amino acids are delicate entities. Most animal protein is cooked, which can denature the amino acids and can make them largely unavailable for our body's use.[7] The Max Planck Institute for Nutritional Research in Germany discovered that cooking destroys about 50 percent of the bioavailability of protein for humans.[8]

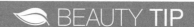

BEAUTY TIP

Vegetarian Doesn't Always Equal Perfect Health

Throughout the book, I speak about the benefits of a plant-based diet and encourage limiting animal protein. But being a vegetarian does not *automatically* mean that you are at the peak of health. You're better off being an omnivore who eats a wide variety and a copious amount of fresh fruits and vegetables than a person who gives up meat altogether and eats poor vegetarian choices, like refined sugars and processed foods. There are some people who eat a small amount of fish and other animal products and consume more greens and fruit than some vegetarians, particularly those who eat mostly refined carbs, like pasta or muffins. These greens- and fruit-eating nonvegetarians are, in fact, better off. Getting some of the good stuff on a regular basis, even if there are also some not-so-ideal foods in the diet, will still drastically increase your health, beauty and vitality. Remember, health is not an all-or-nothing game.

Plant Protein Powder

Raw hemp protein powder and hemp seeds (a nondrug, non-THC variety of hemp and not the one you may be thinking of!) can be found in health food stores. A thirty-gram serving of the powder contains fourteen grams of fiber and eleven grams of protein, and is a better choice than the highly refined and processed soy and whey protein powders. It can be taken straight with water or with almond milk. (I don't recommend putting it in the Green Smoothie, since that would be a protein and fruit combination.)

Even if one wanted to put up an argument for eating animal protein, the meat would have to be eaten raw, the way wild animals eat it. They do not heat it over a fire and cook it until it changes color from pink to dark brown. Dark brown flesh is destroyed and denatured protein. Logically speaking, we can see that this is *not* the matter that builds vibrant, beautiful new tissue!

The truth of the matter is that there is an abundance of *usable* amino acid content found in plants and we do not need to seek out protein from concentrated animal protein sources to make sure we are getting enough. The American Dietetic Association states that "plant protein can meet protein requirements when a variety of plant foods is consumed" and "research indicates that an assortment of plant foods eaten over the course of a day can provide all essential amino acids and ensure adequate nitrogen retention and use in healthy adults; thus, complementary proteins do not need to be consumed at the same meal."[9]

Vegetarianism is supported by the American Heart Association, the American Cancer Society, and the Physicians Committee for Responsible Medicine. For those of us eating *real* plant food—greens, other veggies, sprouts, fruit, seeds and nuts—in abundance, protein deficiency is not a problem. Athletes can supplement their diet with hemp protein, chlorella, hemp seeds and other concentrated forms of plant protein if they are interested in getting a larger dosage of protein.

We just discussed how denatured animal protein's amino acids become toxic and unusable material that the body has to contend with and break down. But that is only the beginning. Animal protein is the most complex of all foods: it takes about twice as long as other foods to pass through our digestive system.[10] As you know from earlier chapters, this provides plenty of time for it to bake in our system into toxic, putrefied sludge as it sucks more of our Beauty Energy!

Moreover, the digestion of meat leaves a large amount of acidic residue in our bodies, including uric acid, purines and ammonia by-products. Let's also not forget the extremely unhealthy and unbalancing overgrowth of *unfriendly* bacteria in our colon, which comes about as a result of the putrefaction process from digesting excess animal proteins.

What about our skin? As mentioned in Chapter 1 (page 5), ammonia not only contributes to an overly acidic condition in the body, but it may be associated with free radical damage, which can lead to fine lines and eventually deep wrinkles. *Eating an abundance of animal protein does not support our skin and beauty. It leaves an acidic residue that ages us.*

There definitely have to be limits to the amount of concentrated protein we consume. The "eat as much protein as you can" mentality that we have been led to adopt is actually quite

True Beauty Story

PETER MORRISON IS A CLIENT OF MINE IN HIS EARLY FIFTIES. AN EX-ATHLETE, HE IS in Gold's Gym nearly every day pumping iron. Over the years, he slowly but surely packed about thirty pounds onto his belly and started developing problems with his heart and thyroid, for which he was on several medications.

When I looked at his diet, sure enough, he had some form of animal protein at every meal, which included egg whites, tuna, steak, chicken and turkey. We changed over to the Glowing Green Smoothie for breakfast and made lunch and dinner salad based. He started eating lots of avocados, sprouts, some nuts and seeds, and kept a small amount of fish and eggs in his diet (around three meals a week). Though he was concerned that his performance in the gym would decline, he was even more concerned about getting healthy for his own sake, as well as the sake of his wife and three children.

In four months he trimmed down from a size thirty-eight waist to a size thirty-two. The puffiness under his eyes disappeared, and the deep furrowed wrinkles across his forehead lightened. His baby face came shining through, and he now looks at least ten years younger! The best news of all? He called me one day, absolutely thrilled to report that he was feeling stronger, had a lot more energy, and was lifting the same amount of weights he had when he was thirty pounds heavier and eating animal protein at every meal! He was strong like the plant-eating gorilla! He was much more toned and he loved his new body, sans belly. We'd cleansed away all that sludge in his body, which was constricting oxygen flow to his muscles. Now not only is he lifting like a champ, but he is eating like a true champ of health.

aging—and dangerous. Taking in more protein than is needed places a heavy burden on our body, creating acidity and wasting Beauty Energy…the very thing we are trying to avoid.

BEAUTY RULES FOR EATING ANIMAL PROTEIN

We have established that we don't need to eat animal protein for nutrition. But many people love eating meat, and you may not want to become a full vegetarian and give up eating meat altogether. That is okay, so long as you stick to these tips when you consume animal protein:

1 | **Buy organic, hormone-free meat, preferably from a local farm or source.** The ugly truth is that factory-farmed animals are fed copious amounts of chemicals, hormones, antibiotics and steroids before being slaughtered, and all these toxins wind up on your plate. A report in 2001 by the Union of Concerned Scientists, co-authored by Margaret Mellon, Ph.D., J.D., director of the organization's Food and Environment Program, examined the use of antibiotics in farmed animals. In a press statement Dr. Mellon said, "Our report finds that there are twenty-five million pounds of antibiotics used in cattle, swine and poultry for nontherapeutic purposes, including growth promotion and disease prevention. The breakdown is about four million pounds in cattle, almost eleven million pounds in swine and ten million pounds in poultry. By contrast, the report finds only three million pounds of antibiotics are used in human medicine. That means we are using eight times the amount of antibiotics in healthy animals as we are using to treat diseases in our children and ourselves."[11]

Remember that *we* also ingest the medications and chemicals that the animals we eat have in them. That is not even to mention the inhumane conditions of these farms, and the despicable and violent manner in which the animals are treated. Purchase only organic, hormone-free animal products at the market, and patronize restaurants that use only these sources.

2 | **Animal protein should be eaten only once a day at most, at dinnertime. Eventually, our goal should be to limit the consumption of meat to two to three times per week at most.**
Eating meat protein a maximum of once a day will provide our bodies with the energy to efficiently digest the more complex protein chains. As you learned with Beauty Food

Pairing, only one kind of animal protein should be eaten at a time. Following the principle of eating Light to Heavy, avoid eating animal protein until dinner so that your Beauty Energy is not wasted during the day and can be freed up for cleansing, weight loss and creating beauty.

And it is important for our health goals to limit meat consumption to only a few times a week, at most.

3 | Animals from the sea, such as sustainable varieties of fish, are preferable to land animals.

Land animals, such as cows, deer, pigs, chickens, etc., tend to have tougher muscle than sea animals and are more difficult to digest, leaving more acidic residue in the body. Fish and other seafood are better choices.

What Does "Free-Range" Really Mean?

We see more and more animal products labeled "free-range," which paints a nice picture of happy chickens sunning in an open field and cows grazing in huge pastures. But does it mean there is less cruelty in the way the animals are handled?

The U.S. Department of Agriculture's Food Safety and Inspection Service (FSIS) requires that chickens raised for their meat have access to the outside in order for a farm to receive the free-range certification.[12] However, the USDA regulations do not specify the quality or size of the outside range or the duration of time an animal must have access to it.[13]

In an interview with CNN in 2004, Richard Lobb, spokesperson for the National Chicken Council, admitted, "Even in a free-range type of style of production, you're basically going to find most of them inside the grow out facility."[14] In a *Washington Post* *Magazine* article in 1995, the author asserted that in the case of birds, the term "free-range" "doesn't really tell you anything about the [animal's] quality of life, nor does it even assure that the animal actually goes outdoors."[15]

The USDA has no specific definition for "free-range" when it comes to beef, pork and other non-poultry products.[16] Farmers do not have to meet any specifications as to the size of the range nor the amount of space given to each animal to call it free-range and "free-range" labeling is unregulated. The USDA relies "upon producer testimonials to support the accuracy of these claims."[17]

The bottom line is that the label "free-range" is essentially meaningless. The best bet for humanely raised meat is to buy from a local farm where you can be sure of how the animals are raised.

This is not to say that you should go out and pile your plate high with seafood every day. Fish is cited as one of the most polluted foods we can eat, as hydrocarbon pollution can concentrate in fish. Two of the biggest water contaminants that lodge in fish are PCBs and mercury. For these reasons, fish and other seafood, while less acid-forming than land animals, should be consumed a maximum of twice per week.

4 | **Be sure to exercise proper Beauty Food Pairing.**
Since protein is already so difficult to digest, meat should not be eaten at the same time as complex starches and carbohydrates. Instead, start with a large green salad and eat your meat along with lots of vegetables.

BEAUTIFUL PLANT-BASED PROTEIN

There's a wide variety of plant-based sources of amino acids and protein:

1 | **Greens and Other Vegetables**
Greens are packed with easily assimilated amino acids. Besides our green drinks, we must also strive to eat vibrant, raw salads made of leafy greens every day.

When we compare calories to protein content, per one hundred calories, broccoli has 11.2

Meat—Not Beautiful for the Planet

A 2006 report from the Food and Agriculture Organization of the United Nations (FAO) cited livestock production as "one of the top two or three most significant contributors to the most serious environmental problems, at every scale from local to global."[18]

Among many of its shocking findings and summaries, the FAO reported that livestock production accounts for 18 percent of global greenhouse gas emissions, which is more than all the world's cars and SUVs combined! And 2.4 billion tons of CO_2 emissions from livestock are a result of the deforestation of over 7.4 million acres of land for pastures and feed-crop fields each year. The livestock sector is the leading contributor to water pollution in the form of nitrogen and phosphorous in the United States, and a large amount of pesticides and antibiotics end up in the water thanks to large-scale livestock production. A third of fossil fuel consumption in the United States is directly related to animal agriculture.

If we really want to be "green," it is essential to look at the environmental impact of what we are choosing to put on our plate three times a day, every day.

grams of protein, as compared with steak, which only has 5.4 grams. Romaine lettuce has 11.6 grams of protein per one hundred calories.[19] Calorie for calorie, plant food has almost *twice* as much protein as meat. Sure we have to eat a greater volume of plant food, but that is a good thing—the more plant foods we eat, the more nutrients and fiber we'll get. Not so with animal protein!

2 | Nuts and Seeds

Raw nuts and seeds are a great source of protein. Nuts are a highly concentrated and calorically dense food, so we need to balance them by making sure we eat some greens and raw veggies before them and along with them. Two to three ounces is a maximum daily amount. If you are an active person or an athlete, or are trying to gain/maintain weight, the portion size can be adjusted slightly higher.

Nuts and seeds must always be eaten

Toxic Body, Toxic Mind

When an animal is about to be slaughtered, it is filled with terror. In this moment of terror the animal's adrenal glands, which are caplike organs located on the top of the kidneys, pour out the stress hormone adrenalin, which flows into the bloodstream and all around its body.

Is it a stretch to believe that when we eat meat, we are taking in some of the adrenalin and immense fear, anger and suffering the animal experienced at slaughter?

The mind and the body are intrinsically connected, and the food we eat has a direct impact on our minds. The more we eat meat, the more anxious, angry, stressed, agitated and nervous we may become. Conversely, the more vegetarian our diet becomes, the more calm, even-keel, clear, joyful, happy, balanced and present we become, and the better we deal with stress and problems. The best proof of this is personal experience!

raw. Roasting alters some of the nuts' beneficial qualities, and commercially packaged seeds and nuts are sometimes cooked in hydrogenated oils, which are full of unhealthy trans fats, and salted. It's best to purchase your seeds and nuts in their natural form.

We should eat cashews in strict moderation or avoid them altogether. Always purchase organic, high quality cashews. While they are great to use in certain recipes, unfortunately, cashews are more susceptible to accumulating various potentially toxic molds (which could be why so many people are allergic to them). They are usually steamed to remove their tough outer shell, so technically they are rarely truly raw, and therefore are not sproutable and shouldn't be soaked. Don't worry, though. There are lots of other healthy nuts to choose from instead! Always store nuts and seeds in the fridge for maximum freshness.

SOAKING NUTS AND SEEDS

Always soak nuts and seeds in water before eating them. Nuts and seeds have inhibitor enzymes on their surface to protect them from germinating until it's safe to do so. Soaking helps deactivate the inhibitor enzymes so that the nutrients are more readily available. Soaking also activates beneficial enzymes and helps convert many of the stored nutrients from a dormant to an active and available state. If you do *not* soak your raw nuts and seeds they will be more acid-forming in the body. Roasted nuts and seeds cannot be soaked.

HOW TO SOAK NUTS AND SEEDS

Place the nuts or seeds in a container and cover with one to two inches of water. The harder the consistency of a nut or seed, the longer you need to soak it. For instance, hard nuts such as almonds require at least twenty-four hours; medium-density nuts such as walnuts or Brazil nuts require around six hours; and soft nuts, such as pine nuts and macadamia nuts, require only two hours or less. Soak seeds like sunflower seeds and pumpkin seeds overnight. The nuts and seeds will plump up as they absorb the water. If soaking nuts or seeds overnight, you should rinse them off before using them. They can stay totally submerged in water for up to two days in the fridge.

I often throw a bunch of different nuts into a bowl and let them soak overnight to save time. If you want the nuts to be totally dry for a certain recipe or to snack on, you can dehydrate them after soaking.

Best Beauty Nuts and Seeds

Almonds	Coconuts	Pecans	Sesame seeds
Brazil nuts	Filberts	Pine nuts	Sunflower seeds
Chia seeds	Hemp seeds	Pumpkin seeds	Walnuts

3 | **Chlorella and Spirulina**

Chlorella, a form of green algae, is about 65 percent protein. There are about fifteen grams of protein in a tablespoon. Two tablespoons a day would supply about thirty grams of protein for those of us who are transitioning or want a diet higher in protein. Spirulina, a blue-green algae, is about 60 percent protein, but since it is less dense, we would have to consume larger quantities of it to get the same grams of protein as in chlorella.

Spirulina and chlorella are both algaes that contain all the essential amino acids and are high in chlorophyll. Both of these algaes are considered a tonic and rejuvenator of the body. They are great to take in powdered or pill form when traveling, when fresh greens are not readily available. They can be helpful in warding off energy slumps and, thanks to their high protein content, they are useful for active athletes.[20] They are also packed with vitamins and minerals. Spirulina is rich in gamma-linolenic acid (GLA), B vitamins, omega-3 fatty acids and enzymes.

If you are an athlete or are on the go, I recommend taking chlorella tablets after a workout or keeping them in your purse or carry-on bag. Chewing these tablets will temporarily satisfy your hunger and provide you with pure protein and necessary minerals. They are perfect on the go, when it is difficult to find high-quality food.

4 | Legumes and Beans

Legumes and beans are an inexpensive protein source that is great for the transitional diet, especially during the Blossoming Beauty phase, and for anyone switching to a vegetarian diet. They have favorable qualities, such as a high protein content and an abundance of certain minerals, vitamins and phytonutrients. But unless we consume the raw sprouted varieties instead of the fully cooked ones, I put legumes and beans in fourth place, after the three plant-based protein categories discussed in the preceding pages.

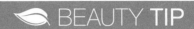

BEAUTY TIP

Pass on the Peanuts

Peanuts are technically a legume, though most people think of them as a nut. I purposely left peanuts off the list of recommended legumes (page 96), because they are prone to mold and fungi. This may be why so many people have allergic reactions to them. Nonorganic peanuts are among the most pesticide-saturated foods in the Western diet.

A study in 1993 found that there were twenty-four different types of fungi that colonized inside of peanuts, even after sterilizing their exterior.[21] A toxic mold called aflatoxin tends to contaminate peanuts, as demonstrated in studies in England[22] and at MIT.[23] In 1988 the International Agency for Research on Cancer (IARC) placed aflatoxin B_1 on the list of human carcinogens, and aflatoxin is considered a potent chemical carcinogen twenty times more toxic than DDT. A number of epidemiological studies were done in Asia and Africa that demonstrated a positive association between dietary aflatoxins and liver cell cancer.[25]

Why take the risk? I recommend sticking to organic, raw almond butter and other varieties of nut butters, and avoiding peanuts altogether.

Why? First of all, they are nature's "oops!" in that they contain *both* protein and starch. (I discuss them here, but they could just as easily be classified with the starches.) Because they incorporate both classes of food, they are difficult to digest—which is exactly why they cause bloating, burping, flatulence, abdominal discomfort and a feeling of heaviness. These are signs that a single food can cause a traffic jam! I do not consider beans a beauty enhancing food and I rarely eat them myself.

Still, legumes and beans are great for the transition diet and are okay enjoyed occasionally. Below is a list of some common ones, but there are many other varieties. Be sure to always buy the whole dried varieties and prepare them yourself. They taste better and you will also avoid any potential metals, chemicals and preservatives that are found in canned beans. It is very important to soak beans overnight to help them digest better.

Best Beauty Legumes and Beans

Adzuki beans	Garbanzo beans (chickpeas)	Kidney beans	Mung beans
Black beans	Great northern beans	Lentils	Navy beans
Black-eyed peas	Green peas	Lima beans	Pinto beans

AVOID (MOST) SOY PRODUCTS

Chances are, in some form or another, we have all heard that soy is a "miracle" food that is a great alternative protein source. The growing soy industry would love to have us all believe that. But the truth is soy may *not* be the miracle health food we have all been led to believe it is.

"Wait!" you say. "What about all the healthy Asians that consume soy?" The truth is that Asians do *not* consume the enormous amount of soy that we consume, but rather use soy as a side dish to rice, vegetables, and small quantities of fish and meat. Furthermore, Asians do *not* consume all the highly processed soy protein isolates and concentrates that are most popular in our country today.

Soy protein isolates are common ingredients in protein powders and packaged food and energy bars. These isolates undergo extensive heat processing in large commercial labs, processing that usually includes acid washing in aluminum tanks and spray drying at high temperatures. To produce textured vegetable protein (TVP), a common ingredient found in processed vegetarian food, high-temperature processing is also necessary.

Let's explore some of the major problems with soy:

1 | The majority of soy in our country is genetically engineered.[26] Genetic engineering greatly alters the nutrient chemistry in certain foods. We want to avoid genetically modified organisms (GMOs)! Genetically engineered soy is reported to have 29 percent less choline, a mineral needed for the development of our nervous system, and 200 percent more lectin, which is associated with food sensitivities.[27] This could be why soy is now one of the top ten allergenic foods in America.

2 | Soy contains trypsin inhibitors. Trypsin is an enzyme that is needed to digest and assimilate protein properly. Trypsin inhibitors may reduce protein digestion and amino acid uptake.[28]

3 | Soy depresses our thyroid function. Soy also contains isoflavones, which are substances that have been shown to depress thyroid function.[29] The thyroid controls the metabolism, among other essential processes in the body, and slowing it down contributes to weight gain. One study showed that genistein in soy foods can cause irreversible damage to enzymes that synthesize thyroid hormones.[30]

ABC's *20/20* did an investigative report on the health claims of soy in June 2000.[31] As part of the investigation, *20/20* cited a letter by Daniel Doerge and Daniel Sheehan, two of the Food and Drug Administration's experts on soy, who stated that "there is abundant evidence that some of the isoflavones found in soy, including genistein and equol, a metabolize of daidzen, demonstrate toxicity in estrogen sensitive tissues and in the thyroid. This is true for a number of species, including humans."[32]

4 | Soy is filled with phytoestrogens. Phytoestrogens are substances that can mess with our endocrine system and can cause a whole list of hormonal complications.[33]

Soy is not good for infants, either. A study published in the *New Zealand Medical Journal* estimated that the phytoestrogens in one day's worth of soy infant formula are the equivalent (on a body weight basis) of five birth control pills.[34]

Say NO to GMOs

Genetically engineered foods are also known as GMOs, or genetically modified organisms. When genes are tampered with in foods, this can cause unanticipated side effects, including an increase in toxins and allergic reactions, and a decrease in nutritional value. Genetic engineering can also upset the delicate balance of our ecosystem and food chain, threatening different plant and animal species on our planet.

A segment of ABC's *Good Morning America* on August 21, 2006, reported that a whopping 75 percent of all processed food in the United States contained ingredients from genetically modified crops.[35] This same segment reported that "the food industry says if the product has corn or soybeans in it—and most processed foods do—it's probably been genetically modified."[36]

How can we avoid these scary pseudo-foods and ingredients? The first thing to do is to avoid processed foods as much as possible. This includes everything from frozen dinners to commercial snack foods, such as all the zillions of varieties of chips that are out there. Secondly, buy organic as much as you can. Organic foods are GMO-free and do not contain artificial pesticides and fertilizers. Since soy and corn are mostly genetically modified, check labels to be sure that these foods are not on the ingredients list. There are other sneaky names they go by. A few of their aliases are dextrin, corn flour, cornmeal, starch, crystalline fructose and textured vegetable protein.

5 | **Soy is one of the foods most heavily contaminated with pesticides.** When we eat plants sprayed with pesticides, we inevitably ingest the pesticides, too.

Pesticides are neurotoxins designed to kill living creatures. There are many cited negative effects of pesticides on humans, which may include damage to the nervous system, reproductive system and particular organs; immune dysfunction; a disruption of hormone function; and developmental and behavioral abnormalities. The more we avoid pesticide-sprayed crops, the better off we will be!

SOY YOU *CAN* EAT

Fermented organic soy products, like miso, tempeh and natto, are acceptable to eat. The long process of fermentation (similarly to how fermentation converts grain to alcohol) deactivates the trypsin inhibitors in soy in a way that cooking cannot and makes these products more easily digestible. Nama shoyu can be consumed in moderation, as it is a "raw" unpasteurized soy sauce made of fermented soybeans. However, nama shoyu contains gluten. Low-sodium tamari, which is gluten and wheat free, is also a great alternative. Bragg Liquid Aminos is a gluten-free, certified non-GMO product that is made of unfermented soybeans but is extremely watered down. For that reason (and because it tastes great!) I do use small amounts of it, as the only real soy product in my diet along with some unpasteurized miso.

Edamame, which are green immature soybeans, contain fewer of the toxins mentioned above, so they can be enjoyed occasionally if you really love them.

For all the reasons cited in the preceding pages, tofu, soy milk, commercial energy bars, soy burgers, soy cheese and other processed products containing soy protein isolates, soy protein concentrate, texturized vegetable protein or hydrolyzed vegetable protein should be avoided! You will be *so* much better off without these products. If you are unsure of a product, check the ingredients list.

THERE IS NOTHING BEAUTIFUL ABOUT DAIRY

I usually stress moderation with all food groups, including fish and other animal protein for those who really want to keep them in their diet. However, this is the one category where there is no room for moderation. No one should eat dairy. Period. We must *all* work to either cut dairy out of our diet immediately or transition it out completely. This is among the first recommendations I make to all my clients that are looking to feel better and become more beautiful. So, in other words…everyone!

You are probably thinking, *Hey, how come I've always heard I should drink milk for calcium? And aren't skim milk and yogurt healthy?* Yes, I would bet that you *have* heard these things because dairy is a big, big business. With hundreds of millions of people consuming dairy every day, there is *a lot* of money to be made by this industry, which in turn also puts a lot of money into guaranteeing that certain health claims are upheld by society, down to providing educational material about the "benefits" of dairy products to children.

From their inception, American dietary guidelines have been influenced by the meat and dairy industries. As Michael Pollan explains in his *In Defense of Food,* when the Senate Select Committee on Nutrition and Human Needs first drafted its dietary guidelines in 1977, the committee intended for Americans to limit red meat and dairy for improved health. But the meat and dairy industries exerted their power and influence to change this, and the committee was forced to compromise by recommending Americans "choose meats, poultry, and fish that will reduce saturated fat intake."[37] Ultimately, both meat and dairy found their prominent place in the food pyramid.

We have always accepted that dairy is simply something humans should consume. After all, it is in every grocery and corner store, and it has always been considered a basic food staple, right? Let's start our dairy discussion by taking a step back and reexamining the issue logically and with an open mind. It's important to understand where dairy comes from, and doing so will help us to see why dairy is not in our best health interests at all.

During the earliest part of life, all mammals drink the milk of their mothers. Baby pigs drink from their mothers, as do baby dogs and cats. Since we are also mammals, we drink the breast milk of our mothers. We are weaned off breast milk within the first few years of our life, and then we shift into eating other foods for the rest of our lives that provide the nutrition necessary for our bodies. This is the natural cycle not only for humans but also for all other mammals on the planet. The natural purpose of cow's milk is to feed baby cows. When the baby cows grow up, they, too, stop drinking milk and shift to eating grass. We are the *only* species on earth that not only refuses to give up milk but furthermore insists on drinking the milk of another species. No adult cows ever drink milk, and adult humans are certainly not meant to be drinking it, either!

As is always the case, when we go against nature's laws, we suffer the consequences. The chemical composition of cow's milk is different from that of human milk, and therefore our bodies are not designed to break it down. Lactase is the enzyme needed to break down and digest the sugar in milk called lactose. Most of our bodies stop or greatly diminish the production of lactase by the time we are two to three years old, as nature did not intend for us to be drinking mothers' milk after that. The devastating consequences of going against nature's innate cycles by continuing to consume dairy include faulty digestion, major sacrifices in Beauty Energy and a myriad of health issues.

THE DANGEROUS PROTEIN IN DAIRY: CASEIN

The common perception is that it is the *fat* in dairy products that is harmful. To avoid the fat, many of us have switched to skim milk, low-fat cheese and fat-free yogurt. But what about the *protein* in dairy?

The main protein in cow's milk is called casein. It makes up 87 percent of cow's milk protein.[38] The other protein in milk is called whey, which makes up a much smaller amount.

There is some casein present in human breast milk, but in cow's milk there is 300 percent more.[39] The casein helps cows develop huge bones. Casein is such a strong binder that it has been used as an ingredient in wood glue.

Without the necessary enzymes such as lactase to break it down, casein coagulates in the stomach and is very difficult for our bodies to break down. This is an enormous waste of Beauty Energy. When casein breaks down in the human stomach, it produces casomorphins, which are peptides, or protein fragments, that have an opioid effect, meaning they act like opiates in the brain, causing a slightly euphoric effect—a troublesome effect considering how unhealthy casein really is! Studies in the 1990s, including one particularly strong one conducted in 1991, hypothesized that casomorphin (from casein) can cause or aggravate autism.[40] Dairy has also been found to *double* the risk of prostate cancer: a Harvard review of research from 2001 found that "men with the highest dairy intakes had approximately double the risk of total prostate cancer, and up to a fourfold increase in risk of metastatic or fatal prostate cancer relative to low consumers."[41]

There are so many thousands of studies on the detrimental effects of dairy that I could go on and on for this entire book. But the strongest argument I can share with you is that of all animal proteins, casein is the one that most consistently and strongly seems to promote cancer. The long-term, in-depth research of *The China Study,* which was funded by such prestigious organizations as the National Institutes of Health, the American Cancer Society and the American Institute for Cancer Research, found a strong correlation between casein intake and the promotion of cancer cell growth when exposed to carcinogens (see more on this topic on page 135). Dr. Campbell, a professor in the Division of Nutritional Sciences at Cornell University, studied the effect of diet on rats exposed to potent carcinogens and found a strong correlation between protein intake and cancer growth. Of all the proteins, Dr. Campbell found that casein most "consistently and strongly promoted cancer" and that it "promoted all stages of the cancer process."[42]

DAIRY CREATES MUCUS, AND MUCUS DEPLETES BEAUTY

Once dairy is put into our body, it becomes an extremely acid-forming food, and as we've learned, acidic foods deplete beauty and encourage weight gain. But dairy has another downside: mucus.

Despite its rather off-putting name, mucus is actually a natural secretion that our body produces to protect the surfaces of membranes. It is clear and slippery, and coats anything we ingest. Where mucus starts to be problematic is when we have too much of it. Mucus engulfs toxins and the toxic remnants of certain foods and can become thick and cloudy to "trap" the toxicity and help it leave the body.[43] Excessive mucus can begin to harden and build up along the walls of our intestines, adding to the sludge and slowing down matter moving through the intestinal tract. Dairy is one of the most mucus-forming foods there is.

When we ingest milk, cheese and other dairy products, it puts a huge burden on the body to try to get rid of the mucus, which wastes a ton of Beauty Energy! Dairy products begin to wreak havoc on our bodies as soon as they are ingested, so our bodies then try desperately to get rid of them in different ways, such as in the form of phlegm, mucus or pimples. Since dairy products are so acid-forming, clogging and difficult to digest, consistently eating them will *not* help us lose the extra weight in those troublesome areas—our bellies, upper arms, thighs, and hips and under our chins. Dairy ultimately keeps us from reaching our true beauty potential.

rBGH AND OTHER UGLY DRUGS

In addition to creating mucus, conventional dairy is packed with hormones and drugs. Dairy cows produce an unnaturally high amount of milk to satisfy commercial purposes. To keep them alive and functioning to accomplish this, they are treated with antibiotics, including penicillin, as well as hormones, like recombinant bovine growth hormone (rBGH). These strong drugs inevitably end up in the milk and make their way into our system.

THE PROBLEM WITH PASTEURIZATION

All commercial dairy products are pasteurized, homogenized and highly processed, meaning they are heated to extremely high temperatures in order to kill any potential bacteria. This processing also kills any natural enzymes that are present in dairy products and makes digesting them even *more* difficult.

We can be sure that any milk or yogurt we get at the grocery store has been pasteurized, otherwise it could not be legally sold. Raw milk and raw cheese (if you have access to them) are better for you than pasteurized milk and cheese, but they still contain casein and are still mucus-forming.

CALCIUM AND OSTEOPOROSIS

We have all heard that we need to consume calcium in order to build strong bones and prevent diseases like osteoporosis. The best way, we have always been told, to get our calcium is from dairy products.

But statistics show that bone issues like osteoporosis and hip fractures are *more* frequent in populations where dairy is *highly consumed* and calcium consumption is generally high.[44] American women drink thirty to thirty-two times as much cow's milk as New Guineans but suffer forty-seven times as many broken hips. An analysis conducted on multiple countries showed a high statistical association between dairy consumption and higher rates of hip fractures.[45] One study out of the Yale School of Medicine in 1992 analyzed the link between protein intake and fracture rates in women fifty years of age and older from sixteen different countries. The study found that the consumption of animal protein was associated with 70 percent of the fractures in the women studied.[46]

Numerous studies show the same correlation: the more protein that is consumed, the more calcium that is lost. One long-term study published in the *American Journal of Clinical Nutrition* found that with seventy-five grams of daily protein intake, more calcium is excreted in the urine than is absorbed into the body, meaning calcium is continually being lost.[47] Even if one's daily dietary calcium intake was as high as fourteen hundred milligrams, this still proved to be true. From his extensive research for the *The China Study*, Dr. T. Colin Campbell reported in the *New York Times* that there was basically no osteoporosis in China, yet the average calcium intake there was 544 mg per day, as compared with 1,143 mg per day in the United States, which was mostly derived from dairy sources.[48]

So what's going on? Cow's milk does in fact have a lot of calcium in it, but much of it is not easily assimilated or used by the body. There is a lot of phosphorus in dairy products, and it binds to the calcium in our

What about Yogurt?

I'm constantly being asked about yogurt. Yogurt is widely advertised as a health food. But let's look at the facts: it contains casein, it is pasteurized and it is mucus-forming. The friendly bacteria in yogurt can easily be had by consuming Probiotic & Enzyme Salad and taking a daily probiotic supplement, which I recommend doing every day. See Chapter 6, Detoxing for Beauty, for more information.

digestive tract and makes most of the calcium impossible to absorb. Plus, as we discussed, dairy products are extremely acidic in the body. As demonstrated by these studies (and additional research cited in the Alkaline-Acid Principle section on page 23), the increased acid load in the body causes us to lose calcium from our bones, since calcium is an alkaline mineral and neutralizes the acidity.

Don't be fooled into looking at a label and being impressed by how much calcium a dairy product contains. Instead, as you shift into a more alkaline state, you'll keep calcium and other alkaline minerals intact in the body. The best sources for calcium are dark, leafy green vegetables, as well as sea vegetables, and nuts and seeds. They are high in calcium and highly alkaline. As we start to cut dairy out of our system, our body will start to clear out the mucus caused by the dairy. Pounds will fall off, our skin will start to clear, and our beauty will start to radiate.

Beautiful Plant Sources of Calcium

Boy choy	Cauliflower	Kale	Sesame seeds
Broccoli	Collard greens	Romaine lettuce	Spinach
Cactus (nopales)	Cucumber	Sea vegetables	Turnip greens

BEAUTIFUL DAIRY ALTERNATIVES

Some of you may be disappointed by this dairy crackdown. I know. Cheese tastes good! I stress the importance of transitioning throughout this book, and part of that is finding alternatives to your favorite foods to make it easier and tastier to eat yourself beautiful.

Cheese lovers, I have great news for you! Goat's milk and goat's cheese are far better options than cow's milk and cow's milk products. The natural enzymes in a goat are far closer to those in humans than those in cows, and we digest goat's milk exponentially better. If you love cheese, you'll be happy to know that you can switch to goat's milk cheese as an occasional treat! It is best to consume goat's milk cheese in its raw, unpasteurized form, though even pasteurized goat's milk cheese is still far better than pasteurized cow's milk products. Sheep's milk cheese is the next best choice.

Here are some healthier foods that mimic your favorite dairy products:

If you like	Try
Milk	Almond milk, hemp milk, rice milk
Cheese	Seed cheese or other non-soy vegan alternatives
	Raw goat's milk cheese or raw sheep's milk cheese (contain lactose)
	Pasteurized goat's milk cheese or pasteurized sheep's milk cheese (not the ideal choice, as the pasteurization makes these products clogging)
	Raw cow's milk cheese (less favorable choice)
Yogurt	Probiotic & Enzyme Salad
	A daily probiotic
	Goat's milk kefir (has clogging properties and is pasteurized)

BEAUTIFUL CARBOHYDRATES AND STARCHES

Carbohydrates, also known as starches or sugars, are a macronutrient that provides us with necessary energy. Many popular diets have demonized carbohydrates and popularized carb counting, but carbohydrates deserve a second chance! We've learned from the Light to Heavy section that starches take less time and energy to digest than protein, and pass through our system much faster. High-quality complex carbs and fruits are perfect for your Beauty Detox.

BEAUTY TIP

Lose the Mind-set that All Carbs Are Bad

Some of us are uneasy about consuming too many starches and are used to counting our calories and carbs. But diets like that are about restriction and often leave us feeling unsatisfied, or thinking about food way too much! The goal with the Beauty Detox is to free up Beauty Energy, speed up digestion and clean out sludge from our system. The high-quality, complex carbs we will be eating on the plan help accomplish all those things and are easily digestible. Refined carbs in the form of refined, processed starch and processed or artificial sugars are completely off the menu.

TYPES OF CARBOHYDRATES

There are three types of carbohydrates: complex, simple and fiber. Complex carbohydrates, also known as starches, include whole, unrefined grains and fiber-rich starches like root vegetables. Simple carbohydrates, also known as sugars, provide the body with fast energy; they include all refined starches and sugars, as well as fruits. Fiber is a kind of complex carbohydrate that is undigested by our bodies. (For more info on the importance of fiber, refer to page 32.) The key to carbohydrates is to eat the correct forms, along with higher quality products.

Natural grain kernels contain the bran, endosperm and germ. Refined carbohydrates—including white-flour breads, pastas and pastries, as well as white rice, potato chips, many breakfast cereals, and most packaged cookies, snacks and baked goods—have been processed to remove the bran and germ. This refinement process removes not only the fiber but also much of the minerals, vitamins and nutrients—in other words, all the good stuff—from the grain! Have you ever noticed how people who eat a lot of refined starch have dry, splotchy skin or pimples? That's because their diets are low in fiber and depleted of minerals. Refined carbohydrates steal our energy and make us feel tired and lazy.

There is a huge difference in the way refined carbohydrates behave in the body compared to unrefined, complex carbs. Complex carbs contain lots of fiber, so it takes longer for our stomach to digest them than refined carbohydrates. This is one instance when slowing things down is a good thing, because it means the glucose is released more slowly and evenly into our bloodstream, satiating us for a longer period of time.

Refined carbohydrates, on the other hand, have little to no fiber, so they cause rapid glucose surges into the bloodstream. This in turn triggers an insulin response from the pancreas to control the level of blood sugar in our bodies, causing swings in our blood-sugar levels—and that energy roller coaster of extreme highs and lows. This pattern can ultimately lead to conditions like type 2 diabetes and high triglyceride levels. Worst of all, refined starches are highly addicting.

In addition to refined starches like white flour, you have to watch out for refined sugars, like sucrose, lactose, brown sugar, molasses, fruit juice concentrates and high fructose corn syrup. Refined sugar is one of the most toxic foods you can eat: it causes extreme energy fluctuations, intense cravings and feelings of depression, anger, anxiety and negativity. High fructose corn syrup is a particularly toxic sugar to avoid. A cheap and highly processed sweetener derived from corn, high fructose corn syrup (HFCS) began replacing corn sugar in processed foods, such as soft drinks, breakfast cereals, cookies and many other baked goods, in the 1980s. Similarly to table sugar, HFCS is made up of the sugars fructose and glucose, but the ratios of these sugars have been altered in the refinement process so that the level of fructose is unnaturally high. A study that appeared in the June 2008 issue of the *Journal of Nutrition,* called "Dietary Sugars Stimulate Fatty Acid Synthesis in Adults," concluded that fructose gets converted into fat more quickly than glucose,[49] making HFCS particularly fattening.

A recent study out of Princeton University and published in *Pharmacology, Biochemistry & Behavior* found that high fructose corn syrup causes considerably more weight gain than table sugar. As one of the study's author's, Princeton professor Bart Hoebel, who specializes in the neuroscience of appetite, weight and sugar addiction, explained:

"Some people have claimed that high-fructose corn syrup is no different than other sweeteners when it comes to weight gain and obesity, but our results make it clear that this just isn't true, at least under the conditions of our tests. When rats are drinking high-fructose corn syrup at levels well below those in soda pop, they're becoming obese—every single one, across the board. Even when rats are fed a high-fat diet, you don't see this; they don't all gain extra weight."[50]

Fructose also has potential beauty-busting properties for our skin in the form of oxidative damage. In a lab study researchers found that the group of rats given fructose had more cross-linking changes in the collagen of their skin than the rats that were fed glucose.[51] As we discussed earlier with ammonia in Chapter 1, page 5, cross-linking may lead to wrinkles and other visible signs of aging.

Conclusion? Keep the über-fattening and skin-marring high fructose corn syrup away from your precious body! To lose weight and discover your most beautiful self, avoid all refined starches and sugars. Don't worry. You'll have so many delicious and satisfying complex carbs and fruits to enjoy on the Beauty Detox plan that you won't miss the mood swings, weight gain or energy swings at all!

Avoid Agave

Agave, also called agave syrup and agave nectar, has become increasingly popular as a "healthy" and "low glycemic" sweetener. Today it is found not only in health stores but even in mainstream grocery stores, as well as in energy bars, drinks, other food products, and health and raw food recipes. I used to use it and promote it myself! But now that I have learned more about it and how it is processed, I have cut it out of my diet altogether. You won't find me promoting agave anymore, and it is not listed in any recipes in this book.

It is true that agave nectar is low glycemic, but it also has a fructose content of up to 90 percent! I know. That was a shocking revelation for me, as well. That is actually higher than even high fructose corn syrup, which averages about 55 percent fructose. As Dr. Ingrid Kohlstadt, a fellow of the American College of Nutrition and an associate faculty member at the Johns Hopkins School of Public Health, points out "Agave is almost all fructose, a highly processed sugar with great marketing."[52]

Agave syrup, or agave nectar, is not a whole food found in nature. Instead it usually has to undergo extensive processing to arrive at that sweet liquid syrup form, and this may involve many chemicals and/or heating processes, even if the agave syrup is labeled "raw."[53]

This is all very disappointing, because agave is so convenient to use in desserts and other recipes. But fructose is fructose. Period. And it is certainly not worth the health risks. The best sweetener to use is stevia, which you can buy in a powdered or a concentrated liquid form. (Some people find it bitter at first, but your taste buds adapt. I used to think that also, but now I don't notice any bitterness at all!)

Here is a list of a few other sweetener choices, which should be used in strict moderation: Dried fruit, such as figs and dates, can be used as sweeteners when blended in certain recipes. Raw honey contains fructose, but it is a whole, natural food (though not vegan). Be sure to purchase only raw honey that is organic, and if possible purchase locally from a beekeeper who uses ethical practices. Organic, pure maple syrup is another choice when you need a liquid sweetener. It is not raw, because it undergoes heat processing, and it is made up of sucrose, but it doesn't require as much processing as agave and artificial sweeteners and is a much better choice. Xylitol, a low-glycemic substitute that is actually a sugar alcohol naturally occurring in the fibers of fruits and vegetables, is also an acceptable option.

AVOIDING GLUTEN FOR BETTER BEAUTY

Contrary to popular belief, "whole-wheat" bread, bagels, crackers and other products are *not* so beautiful for the body. While wheat is an ancient crop, the wheat we farm today is hardly what wheat once was in its original form. Today wheat is grown in mineral-depleted soil and is heavily sprayed with pesticides and other chemicals. Some of the scary chemical fungicides, insecticides and herbicides that it is dosed with include disulfoton (Di-Syston), methyl parathion, chlorpyrifos, dimethoate, dicamba and glyphosate.[54]

Though these substances are approved and recognized as "safe" for commercial crop use, we definitely want to reduce all exposure to these potentially beauty-squashing toxic chemicals, which find their way into our body through the wheat and wheat-based products we eat. Moreover, despite all these toxic pesticides, wheat can be stored for long periods in silos and can often be contaminated to varying degrees with molds and fungi, which add to the sludge and steal our Beauty Energy. Wheat is one of the eight most common foods—the others are milk, eggs, peanuts, tree nuts (like cashews), fish, shellfish and soy—and these account for about 90 percent of all allergic reactions in the United States.[55] What makes wheat so allergenic is the gluten present in it, which is its primary protein. Gluten, which is also present in rye and barley, can cause toxic reactions that trigger our immune system and may cause inflammation of the intestinal tract.

Many of us may have an intolerance to gluten and may not even be aware of it or experience any overt symptoms. But James Braly, M.D., and Ron Hoggan, M.A., coauthors of the book *Dangerous Grains: Why Gluten Cereal Grains May Be Hazardous to Your Health,* claim that gluten intolerance is a factor not only in celiac disease (an autoimmune disease in which the lining of the small intestine is damaged and cannot process gluten) but also in many autoimmune disorders and neurological and psychiatric conditions, including rheumatoid arthritis, hyperthyroidism and liver disease.[56]

Eliminating highly and commonly allergenic foods, such as gluten, from our diets can help improve our overall health, help eliminate sugar and carb cravings, help stabilize our moods and help us lose weight. You may not feel results immediately when you go gluten-free, because it can take some time for any inflammation to go down. But over time, you'll notice the positive difference.

I have seen these positive effects in so many of my clients, but I've also experienced them for myself. Since cutting out gluten, I have noticed that my energy level has improved and my weight has stabilized—and I don't crave bread at all anymore!

To achieve your highest level of beauty, work towards cutting out all wheat products, including cereals, pastries, pasta, breads, pretzels, cookies, bagels and the like. Now, don't freak out! It doesn't mean you'll never eat a piece of bread again for the rest of your life. You'll just replace wheat and wheat products with much higher quality grains.

STARCHY VEGETABLES: A BEAUTIFUL CHOICE

Starchy vegetables are an excellent addition to a meal, and they taste great and definitely satisfy your hunger. There are so many incredible starchy vegetables and tubers out there. Have fun looking into varieties that you don't already know about. There's yuca, spaghetti squash, acorn squash, kabocha squash, butternut squash and many more.

The best way to eat these starchy vegetables is to cook them well; in this case they digest better that way and taste better, too. Yams, winter squash and sweet potatoes can be thoroughly baked at high temperatures. Winter squash is excellent cooked, then pureed as soup.

Best Beauty Starchy Vegetables

Red jacket potatoes	Squash, all varieties	Sweet potatoes	Yams

BEAUTY GRAINS

The four best Beauty Detox grains are millet, quinoa, amaranth and buckwheat. These grains are gluten-free, and all except for buckwheat, also known as kasha, (which leaves a slightly acid-forming residue) digest to leave a slightly alkaline residue in the body. You should always eat veggies first and along with grains to control portion size. Still, these grains add important fiber and help stop cravings for refined carbs, like breads and pastries.

Even though you may not have ever eaten these grains in the past, they are generally easy to find: quinoa is even sold at stores like Trader Joe's and the "ethnic" section of your

Beauty Grains and Starches

BEST BEAUTY CHOICES	
Amaranth	Quinoa
Buckwheat (also called kasha)	Soba noodles (made of buckwheat)
Millet	Starchy vegetables (winter squash, yams, sweet potatoes, etc.)

NEXT BEST BEAUTY CHOICES	
Beans, all varieties	Chickpeas
Black-eyed peas	Gluten-free crackers, pastas and other foods
Brown or wild rice	Lentils

WORST BEAUTY CHOICES—AVOID THESE	
Processed and refined starches and sugars	Wheat and wheat products
Rye and barley	White rice

local grocery store. They are very inexpensive (a pound of millet is around two or three dollars), easy to cook and prepare, and make delicious accompaniments to veggies and salads to add some density to meals. Products made from these grains are also available, including millet bread, millet cereal, kasha cereal, quinoa crackers, quinoa pasta, quinoa flakes and cream of buckwheat cereal. In fact, you'll find that it's easy enough to swap these grains for your current starch staples, like rice and pasta. When you switch to these grains and grain products, you will not miss anything! That is, except for the excess pounds.

It is important to soak grains at least eight hours, and preferably overnight. This will help deactivate the enzyme inhibitors that coat all grains (and beans) and will make them even easier to digest. Get in the habit of planning ahead. Soak some quinoa or millet the night before, and make enough to last you for a couple of days or to pack for lunch.

The reality is that sometimes we might have trouble finding certain products, like millet bread, when we eat in restaurants or when we are traveling. The key in these situations is to do your best! Rice is a better alternative to wheat, and brown rice is a better choice than refined white rice. Anytime we eat a grain or starch product, and especially when we eat these less than ideal grain or starch products, we should take a digestive enzyme to help them digest better. (See Chapter 6, Detoxing for Beauty, for more information on enzymes.) And remember, it is the norm, not the occasional exceptions to the rule, that really counts.

CHOOSE BEAUTY FATS AND EAT IN MODERATION

Fat should be limited in our diet. While fat has some important functions, such as helping to make our skin supple and beautiful, lubricating our joints, strengthening our cell membranes against oxidation damage, and helping to protect and insulate our nervous system, we will be getting enough fat naturally from our diet, in the form of avocados, seeds and nuts, so that we do not have to supplement or seek it out.

There are many different types of fat:

○ Saturated fats: Found in meat and dairy products, as well as some plant sources, like coconut oil.

BEAUTY TIP

The Glycemic Index

Over the past few decades the glycemic index (GI) has become a bit of a buzzword. The GI is a measure of the effect of a particular food on your blood sugar.

But the GI is not the only deciding factor on whether a food is healthful or not. Certain foods, like bananas, papayas, apricots and carrots, have a higher GI number, but they are still natural, healthy foods. We don't want to eat a diet loaded with *all* high-glycemic foods, but some nutrient-dense foods that have a higher GI, such as some fruits and vegetables, are healthy and have lots of plant fiber. A diet loaded with dietary fiber that includes fruits, vegetables and certain natural, unrefined whole-grain carbohydrates will help stabilize blood sugar levels. In fact, some researchers believe that it is the presence or lack of *plant fiber* that is the most reliable indicator of blood glucose control.[57]

The bottom line is this: we will reach our ultimate health and beauty goals by eating a diet filled with nutrient- and fiber-rich foods in their natural, unrefined and unprocessed state.

- ○ Unsaturated fats: Often referred to as "heart-healthy fats," these are found in plant sources, like avocados, nuts, seeds and olive oils, as well as in fish.

- ○ Trans-fatty acids: Unsaturated fats that have been altered through the process of hydrogenation. Considered the worst kind of fat, trans fats have been associated with heart disease and other health issues. These types of fats are extremely harmful to our health and beauty and should be avoided in all quantities!

Fatty acids are the main building blocks of fats. Just as there are eight essential amino acids, there are two essential fatty acids that must come from foods: omega-3 and omega-6 fatty acids. Most people get too much omega-6 fatty acid, which is present in foods like vegetable oils and margarine, but not enough omega-3. I recommend adding one tablespoon a day of ground flaxseed to your salad, which will supply your daily dosage of omega-3 essential fatty acids. We need these for proper brain and nerve functioning.

Okay, enough with the technicalities. Here's the deal: if your goal is to lose weight, it is a good idea to cut back on oil, even healthy oil. Oil is extremely dense and loaded with calories, so it can really plump us up. In recent years the media has popularized the consumption of certain plant oils, like olive oil, as a good source of healthy unsaturated fat. But oil is still oil, no matter how you slice it—or, in this case, pour it! I have included several oil-free salad dressings in the recipe section. If you want to lose weight, limit oil in your diet (though if you are naturally very thin, keeping some oil in your diet will help keep your weight up). I stopped adding olive oil to my salads years ago.

As you learned in Chapter 3, Eating for Beauty, a *large* amount of fat should never be eaten with protein—that is an improper Beauty Food Pairing. Significant amounts of fat, and especially refined and heated fat, delay the secretion of hydrochloric acid, which is needed for efficient protein digestion in our stomach. If you are planning a fish, chicken or other animal protein-based dinner, I would recommend omitting the oil from your pre-dinner salad. Digestive enzymes high in lipase should be taken while consuming fats other than avocados. (See Chapter 6, Detoxing for Beauty, for more on this.)

IDEAL SOURCES OF PLANT-BASED FAT

Avocados: Technically a fruit, avocados are a wonderful source of fat for your Beauty Detox. Dr. Norman Walker calls avocados "just about the finest fat we can put in our bodies." With their creamy texture and beautifying oils, avocados are extremely filling and provide long-burning fuel. I have found them essential in my own diet, as they provide heaviness and help keep me feeling full until dinner. Those used to eating heavier diets will find avocados a savior and a good replacement for meat and dairy products. When we are trying to lose weight, we must limit all fat, so half of a large avocado or one small avocado a day is the maximum amount we should consume.

Avocados contain some water and digest very easily out of the system. That said, when eating avocados, it is best to consider them the concentrated food for Beauty Food Pairing. Eat them with greens or non-starch vegetables, or following other kinds of fruit. For instance, if you are eating a salad for lunch with avocado, avoid eating nuts with it. If you plan on eating a concentrated protein, like some fish at dinner, skip avocados in your green salad. An avocado would be too much fat to eat with protein—that is a combination for poor digestion and weight gain!

When eaten properly, avocados can be one of our best Beauty Detox friends. I personally eat one avocado almost every single day, or one and a half when I am really active. For a quick lunch, I'll layer some avocado slices on a few nori wrappers (the black seaweed that sushi is wrapped in, which you can get at health markets) with sprouts and lots of baby spinach, squeeze some lemon and seasoning on them and wrap them up. A super-easy, filling and healthy lunch made in about one minute!

Other beautifying fatty fruits you can try are durian (an Asian fruit) and olives, but adhere to the same food pairing rules as when eating avocados.

Raw, cold-pressed oils: For certain recipes and dishes, a small amount of oil is allowable. It is best to use unrefined oils that are raw and cold-pressed. The best ones are unrefined coconut oil, flaxseed oil, olive oil, pumpkin seed oil, hemp seed oil, borage seed oil, evening

🍃 BEAUTY TIP

Cook with Coconut Oil

If there is a dish that you would like to cook with a small amount of oil, coconut oil is a great choice because it has a higher smoke point than other oils. In other words, because it is nearly a completely saturated fat, it is much less susceptible to heat-induced damage and will stay stable at higher temperatures. Plus, cooking with it is an easy way to get coconut oil into your diet, along with all of its wonderful beauty and health benefits!

primrose oil and sunflower oil. It is vital that we consume these oils in a totally unrefined state. If they have been refined in some way, which could include processes such as bleaching or deodorizing, these oils are much harder on our liver and lack the essential fatty acids.

Unrefined oils do not contain preservatives and are never exposed to light or oxygen. It is best to purchase them in dark glass bottles, as light can cause oxidation. While they may be pricier than commercial oils, your liver and your skin deserve the best, so consider this an investment in looking and feeling your best!

Coconut oil is a very special oil. It can be consumed in moderation in desserts in its virgin, or unprocessed, form. Coconut oil is easily emulsified during digestion without putting any burden on the liver or gallbladder, so it frees up Beauty Energy. About 50 to 55 percent of the fatty acids in coconut oil are lauric acid, which can actually help support and restore our thyroid. In their book, *Virgin Coconut Oil,* Brian and Marianita Shilhavy point out that while coconut oil is a saturated fat, it is cholesterol free and trans-fatty acid free and has actually been shown to help lower cholesterol levels due to its ability to stimulate thyroid function.[58]

Virgin coconut oil is composed of medium-chain-length fatty acids, or triglycerides (MCTs), which are shown to have many health benefits, including raising the body's metabolism, and acting as an antiviral, antifungal and antibacterial agent. Virgin coconut oil is the best natural source of MCTs besides human breast milk.

Nuts and seeds: We've already discussed raw nuts and nut butters in detail in the protein section, but they also contain healthy beauty fat. Nut and seed pâtés are great staples for heavier meals. Nuts and seeds should always be soaked first and rinsed to remove inhibitor enzymes, which make

Free Radicals and Antioxidants

Free radicals are atoms or groups of atoms that have at least one unpaired electron and become unstable and highly reactive. They are created as a result of the process of oxidation, that is, when a substance combines with oxygen due to a wide variety of internal and environmental stresses, such as exposure to pollution, chemicals and radiation. Free radicals are believed to cause tissue damage at the cellular level—harming our DNA and cell membranes, and accelerating the aging process.

Antioxidants are substances that may protect cells from the damage caused by free radicals by working to stabilize them. Examples of antioxidants include beta-carotene, lycopene and vitamins A, C and E, all of which can be found in plant foods.

them more difficult to digest. Since nuts are already dense and rich in protein and fat, enjoy them as the heaviest food in a meal and do not combine them with avocados or concentrated animal protein of any kind. Check out some of the recipes in Chapter 11.

DESTRUCTIVE COOKED OILS

Cooked oils and fried foods are among the most aging, fattening and acid-forming types of food we can consume. Eating excessive cooked fat can cause acne, premature aging, weight gain, unfavorable body odor, liver stagnation and cardiovascular problems, to name just a few. (That makes that occasional "innocent" pile of fries not so appetizing anymore, huh!?)

Cooked fat clogs the body and makes it very difficult for the body to metabolize, while putting a heavy burden on our liver and digestive system—all of which make us gain excessive weight. Cooking animal oils and animal fat in particular can create oxidation and free radicals associated with the visible signs of aging on our skin, as well as other health issues.

Margarine, hydrogenated oils and trans-fatty acids of all kinds, as well as refined oil, are some of the worst kinds of fat to eat. And saturated fats and dietary cholesterol from animal products should be limited; excessive dietary cholesterol can weaken the liver and is associated with health issues like heart disease and high blood cholesterol levels.

🍃 BEAUTY **TIP**

Eat Your Spotted Bananas!

Fruits that are ripe are alkaline-forming. Organic fruits are the most alkaline, because they are grown in mineral-dense soil. Fruits that are *not* ripe can actually be acid-forming. For example, if you were to test the pH of two different bananas, you would find that the one that has the most black spots has a higher and more alkaline pH than the one with a slightly green top and no black spots! So remember to reach for only ripe fruits to eat or use in your Glowing Green Smoothies.

In addition to being better for you, ripe fruit is also juicier and tastes sweeter. How can we tell when a fruit is ripe? That is, besides the obvious spotted banana? As a fruit ripens, it deepens in color and smells sweet. In general, you should look for an evenly colored and textured fruit with a delicious smell. The color should be bright and full, with no hints of green or white unless the fruit naturally has these colors. With fruits like melons, a discolored area indicates where the fruit rested on the ground, which also happens to be the sweetest and most delicious part of the fruit.

On the contrary, raw, uncooked fat—especially avocados—will *further* our health and beauty. Let's always strive to eat our fats in their natural, unheated and beautifying form.

FRUIT: THE ULTIMATE BEAUTY FOOD

Fruit is the most life-enhancing food we can put into our bodies. It has the highest water content of any of the food groups and supplies us with vital amino acids, minerals, vitamins and fatty acids. Because fruit breaks down the fastest in our system, while leaving no toxic residue, it supplies us with readily available energy that can be used for immediate fuel.

Of all foods, fruit is the strongest cleanser. We can think of fruits as the cleansers for the body and greens and other vegetables as the builders. Fruit helps to dissolve toxic substances and cleanse our tissues and system, stirring up old toxic residue inside of our bodies.

Best Beauty Fruits

Acai berries	Cranberries	Kumquats	Plums
Apples	Cucumbers	Lemons	Pomegranates
Apricots	Currants	Limes	Prunes
Avocados	Figs	Mangoes	Raisins
Bananas	Goji berries	Nectarines	Raspberries
Blackberries	Gooseberries	Oranges	Strawberries
Blueberries	Grapefruits	Papayas	Tangerines
Cantaloupe	Grapes	Peaches	Tomatoes
Cherimoyas	Guavas	Pears	Watermelon
Cherries	Honeydew melon	Persimmons	

Fruit becomes a truly healthy food only when our bodies are alkaline and cleansed enough to handle it, and when we have a good amount of healthy bacteria within to break down the fruit sugar. Many of us have unknowingly compromised our friendly flora with antibiotics, hormonal medications (like birth control pills), preservatives, environmental pollution and many other factors. When you're first beginning your Beauty Detox, you may have an adverse reaction to fruit. If eating fruit causes nausea, burping, bloating or intense stomach upset, you may have an acidic condition in the body or sugar issues that prevent you from metabolizing fruit.

If you are more than fifty pounds overweight, come from a lifestyle of eating devitalized and processed foods *or* suspect you have some kind of candida or yeast imbalance in your body, you should remain in Phase 1, Blossoming Beauty, for one to three months longer than suggested, or until you have become balanced. This phase doesn't include sweet fruits.

Fruits That Are Lower in Sugar

All these fruits have some level of sourness and are good choices for reintroducing fruit into the diet for people who are sensitive to sugar. Avocados, cucumbers and tomatoes are technically fruit, but they are not sweet and thus are also fine.

Blackberries	Grapefruit	Limes
Blueberries	Green apples	Lemons
Cranberries	Kiwis	Pomegranates
Currants	Kumquats	Strawberries

BEAUTY **TIP**

Sexy Seeded Fruits

The very definition of a fruit is that it bears its own seed. These seeds have the DNA programmed in them to become huge trees or plants. Seeded fruits are pregnant with fertility and have the potential to reproduce. Seeded, natural fruit is bursting with life force; when we eat it, we take in that energy and increase our own magnetism.

When a fruit is sold in "seedless" varieties, it means that that particular fruit's genetic makeup has been tampered with by scientists in a lab to produce strains that sell well commercially. Scientists have engineered a way to make these hybrid fruits lack a double set of chromosomes in their reproductive cells. In other words, these fruits don't have seeds and can no longer reproduce—which defies the very definition of what a fruit is in the first place! To make matters worse, hybrid fruit can also be much higher in sugar and lower in minerals.

To feel sexier from within, go for the natural, organic varieties of fruits, which bear their own seeds. I relish picking out about twelve seeds from the lemon squeezer before pouring the juice onto my salads, knowing I am getting the freshest, most natural kind of lemon juice there is to nourish me!

Fruit should be eaten raw. When heated to high temperatures, fruit loses its cleansing properties and many of its nutrients and becomes acidic in the body, rather than alkaline-forming. Cooked fruit and cooked fruit products to avoid include pasteurized juices (pretty much all bottled fruit juices and beverages), jams, jellies, cooked fruit pies and other such desserts, commercial applesauce and other fruit sauces. Dried fruits, such as dried figs (unsulfured, with no sugar added), are concentrated and higher in sugar, so they should be eaten in limited amounts such as in desserts.

What Is Candidiasis and How Do I Know If I Have It?

Candidiasis, or Candida-Related Complex (CRC), is a condition that can develop when there is an overgrowth of the yeast *Candida albicans.* Many different factors cause candidiasis: taking antibiotics, birth control pills or other hormones, or eating excessive amounts of processed foods.

Some of the symptoms include intense cravings for sugar, bread or alcoholic beverages; oppressive menstrual cramps; chronic vaginitis; chronic fungal infections of the skin or nails; long-term insomnia; chronic constipation and/or diarrhea; excessive bloating or intestinal gas; anxiety attacks; excessive emotional outbursts or crying; reoccurring headaches; mental spaciness; food allergies; and extreme difficulty in losing weight.

It is especially common in women—though many women do not even realize they have it. This yeast thrives off sugars, so you have to be very careful about what you eat until you've rid your body of candidiasis. If you even suspect that you may have it, start your Beauty Detox with the Blossoming Beauty phase, which is a no-sugar, no-gluten eating plan that will make your body more alkaline.

There are some lab tests being developed to diagnose candidiasis and other yeast-related conditions. However, the best way to tell whether or not you have candidiasis is your history, your symptoms, and how well you respond to treatment. I have had many, many female clients that had no clue that they had candidiasis but were able to finally lose weight and get their life back after following the Blossoming Beauty phase.

The best way to figure out whether you have candidiasis is to stay strictly in the Blossoming Beauty phase for two weeks and see if your symptoms start to clear up. (If they improve, you've pinpointed the problem, and sticking with Blossoming Beauty for one to three months total will usually clear it up. However, some may need to stay in Blossoming Beauty for even longer and in extreme cases for up to a year. (For more on this, see page 167). By closely adhering to this program, you will starve the yeast and rebalance your body once and for all! If you have had a chronic problem losing weight in the past, this rebalance could really help finally set you back on track for easy weight loss.

BEAUTY GREENS AND VEGETABLES

As we discussed in Chapter 4, Beauty Minerals and Enzymes, greens are our most important food group. Greens are among the most nutrient dense of all foods and are full of alkaline minerals, chlorophyll and amino acids. They make up our key beauty foods that regenerate and purify our cells. We'll be drinking the Glowing Green Smoothie and Glowing Green Juice daily in the Radiant and True Beauty phases.

Besides greens, we want to eat from a wide range of vegetables, which will supply us with key minerals, enzymes and vitamins. Their fiber will help sweep waste from the body, as well as fill us up. All vegetables leave an alkaline residue, with the exception of starchy vegetables (see Beautiful Carbohydrates and Starches on page 105).

It is highly preferable to eat all vegetables fresh. However, frozen vegetables are a good choice if you don't have time to pick up, or don't have access to, fresh produce. Freezing individual portions of the Glowing Green Smoothie or the Glowing Green Juice and thawing them out the night before can be a great time-saver. However, canned vegetables (and anything canned, really!) should be avoided altogether.

RAW VERSUS COOKED VEGETABLES

Eating vegetables raw is key to obtaining the most beautifying vitamins, enzymes and nutrition, so we should be eating plenty of salads and raw veggies every day. Any type of heat will destroy some of their nutrients.

But I know it is not reasonable for all of us to eat only salads all the time! It is okay to have some cooked vegetables, especially when we are transitioning and at dinner. When cooking vegetables, you want to avoid overcooking them, because you want to preserve the nutrients as much as you can. Steaming or lightly sautéing, for example, will retain some of the vegetables' nutrients and ensure they digest easily.

Starchy vegetables are a part of the Beauty Detox Solution eating plan but have different properties than other vegetables. (For more information on them, refer to the Beautiful Carbohydrates and Starches section on page 105.) In contrast to non-starch vegetables, starchy veggies *should* be cooked well.

Best Beauty Greens and Vegetables

Artichokes (Jerusalem)	Collard greens	Parsley
Arugula	Dandelion greens	Parsnips
Asparagus	Dill	Peppers
Bean sprouts (all varieties)	Endive	Radishes
Beet greens	Escarole	Romaine lettuce
Beets	Frisée	Scallions
Bok choy	Green beans	Shallots
Broccoli	Kale	Spinach
Brussels sprouts	Lamb's quarters	Swiss chard
Cabbage (green, red or Chinese)	Leeks	Turnips
Carrots	Lettuce	Watercress
Cauliflower	Mushrooms	Wheatgrass
Celery	Mustard greens	
Chard	Okra	
Chives	Onions	

WHY ORGANIC MATTERS

The only true way to reach our highest and most beautiful potential is to be in harmony with the laws of nature. Mother Nature knows best! Organic farming is completely in line with natural laws and treats the soil and our earth with the respect they deserve. In organic farming, crops are rotated so as not to deplete the soil of its vital minerals. The produce is carefully and thoughtfully grown. Organic crops have the highest energy and life force possible, which are exhibited in a greater vitamin and mineral content than in commercial counterparts, and higher levels of phytochemicals and antioxidants. *Strong, beautiful*

Support Local Farmers' Markets

I know that making the choice to buy organic can be limited by geographic location and budget. We must do the best that we can. If you are limited for either of these reasons, I suggest you look into our local friends—our local farmers! Local farm produce is usually priced pretty competitively with commercial produce. Even though local produce isn't always labeled organic, as it can be pricey to get certified, local farmers are still oftentimes using organic practices! As they operate much smaller farms, they don't have to resort to many of the mass commercial farming practices. If you go to your local farmers' market, you can talk to the farmers about their fertilizer methods and other farming practices. Local *and* organic is by far the best combination.

and chemical-free produce builds strong, beautiful and chemical-free bodies!

Organic farmers allow fruits and vegetables to fully ripen on the vine, instead of relying on combustive chemicals to force them to ripen prematurely and artificially. Once a food is picked, it cannot absorb any more minerals or nutrition from the plant it was picked from, the sun or the soil. It makes total sense that since organic foods are usually picked at later stages and are grown in much better soil, they yield much higher quantities of beautifying vitamins and minerals and their taste is far superior! When I was backpacking for a year and a half through Asia, I was so spoiled by the out-of-this-world flavorful, sweet bananas that grew naturally across the Philippines and Laos. On the polar end of the spectrum are the wimpy-tasting commercial ones that you can buy at gas stations. They taste like something molded into the shape of a banana, but with only a fraction of the flavor added in. So unsatisfying!

A study conducted in 2002 by Rutgers University revealed an astonishing difference in mineral content between organic and conventional produce, especially in terms of the minerals iron, calcium, magnesium, manganese and potassium. The Rutgers research found 87 percent more trace elements and minerals in organic produce versus produce that was commercially grown.[59] These are among our key beauty minerals.

Since the 1950s, as commercial farming has adopted practices like chemical fertilizing and plant breeding, and soil conditions have declined, there has been a marked decrease in the average nutritional content of grains as well as fresh fruits and vegetables.[60] To quote Michael Pollan from *In Defense of Food:*

USDA figures show a decline in the nutrient content of the forty-three crops it has tracked since the 1950s. In one recent analysis, vitamin C declined by 20 percent, iron by 15 percent, riboflavin by 38 percent, calcium by 16 percent. Government figures from England tell a similar story: declines since the fifties of 10 percent or more in levels of iron, zinc, calcium, and selenium across a range of food crops. To put this in more concrete terms, you now have to eat three apples to get the same amount of iron as you would have gotten from a single 1940 apple.[61]

All these commercial farming practices are directly in opposition to the natural laws of growing food and are motivated by the desire to grow more produce faster and sell more at a cheaper cost, yet we're the ones paying for it.

Not only is organic food more nutritious, but it doesn't contain the unhealthy pesticides used in conventional farming. Pesticides are neurotoxins that destroy the central nervous system of various pests. Whenever we eat conventionally grown produce, we invariably eat trace pesticides, as well. Exposure to these pesticides may contribute to a whole host of health problems, such as cancer, birth defects, damage to the central nervous system and developmental problems.[62] These pesticides and herbicide poisons have a serious impact on our beauty, as well: they contribute to toxic sludge and tax our liver. Clean food equals clean bodies, which equal clean, natural beauty. Period.

If you can't buy all organic produce (see the box Foods You Must Buy Organic on page 124), you can look into the various fruit and vegetable cleansers in the produce sections of health food stores. You can soak your produce for thirty minutes to an hour in a mixture of filtered water and ³/₄ cup of apple cider vinegar or one of these produce cleansers. This can at least help with reducing some of the pesticide content, though, of course, this won't help increase the mineral content of produce.

Achieving real beauty is about total harmony with the universe and our earth

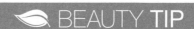

BEAUTY TIP

Look for OceanSolution Produce

A company called OceanSolution created the world's first "mineralizer." As opposed to chemical-filled fertilizer, OceanSolution mineralizer contains every element in its natural proportion to truly nourish the soil and the plants grown in it. OceanSolution is sustainable and renewable. Look for certified and labeled OceanSolution produce in your health or grocery store!

and all the elements that supply us—the sun, water and air—with our foods. Part of this harmony and understanding is that we should never tamper with nature or attempt to improve upon her perfection.

We take a stand for what we believe in by the choices we make and the way we live our life. Choose organic as much as you can and whenever you can. Your beauty and health are definitely worth the investment! When we choose organic, we choose nature, and we become more naturally beautiful ourselves.

Foods You Must Buy Organic

In his book *Diet for a Poisoned Planet,* David Steinman shares his extensive research into which produce has the most toxic residue from conventional farming methods.[63] He analyzed foods for more than one hundred different industrial chemicals and pesticides, and he used laboratory detection limits that were about ten times more sensitive than normal FDA detection standards.

From Steinman's toxicity analysis, he was able to determine which foods were absolutely essential to buy organic. So if you aren't buying *all* organic, always look for organic versions of these foods:

Apples	Celery	Peaches	Raisins	Strawberries
Bell Peppers	Cucumbers	Pears	Spinach	Summer Squash

SPROUTS: A POWERFUL FOOD FOR YOUR BEAUTY DETOX

Spouts are one of the most magical and beneficial foods that we can consume. Seeds have the DNA to continue the next generation and to grow into a plant or a tree. When a seed becomes sprouted, it begins to transition from a dormant seed into an actual living plant. In this exciting process of maturation, much of the stored nutrition begins to multiply. The protein content can increase by up to 30 percent and the enzyme content can increase up to 1,000 percent or more. The availability of chlorophyll, fiber, the B vitamins, as well as vitamins C, E and K will also dramatically increase.

Many health practitioners believe that sprouts are one of the greatest healing foods available. Dr. Ann Wigmore wrote about and researched sprouts extensively, and both the Ann Wigmore Natural Health Institute in Rincón, Puerto Rico, and the Hippocrates Health Institute in West Palm Beach, Florida, which was inspired by Dr. Wigmore's work, stress the importance of consuming sprouts. Many people visit these institutes to heal their bodies naturally of illness, and they are fed a diet high in sprouts.

Cost-wise, I don't think you can find more comprehensive nourishment for less money! You can find containers of sprouts at your local grocery store for no more than a few dollars. If you have the kitchen space and motivation, you can also try sprouting your own seeds. Be sure to add sprouts to your salads, wraps and recipes as much as possible!

BEAUTY SECRET
According to yogic philosophy, sprouts are the highest *prana* (energy) food of all since a sprout is gathering as much energy as possible to transition from a seed to a plant.

Best Beauty Sprouts

Adzuki	Clover	Lentil	Radish
Alfalfa	Cow pea (black-eyed pea)	Millet	Sesame
Broccoli	Fenugreek	Mung	Sunflower (my favorite!)
Cabbage	Green pea	Mustard	Triticale
Chickpea	Kamut	Oat	Watercress

BEAUTY FROM THE SEA

Sea vegetables are a very important beauty food group. You may not have heard a lot about sea vegetables, especially if you've been eating a SAD (Standard American Diet), but these are worth familiarizing yourself with!

Usually when we hear "seaweed" or "sea vegetable," we think exclusively of Japanese food, but sea vegetables have been consumed for thousands of years all around the world, from Australia to the British Isles. Sea vegetables can easily be added into our everyday diets. They are great in salads, pâtés, on vegetables, and in soups. They are extremely rich in vitamins A, B$_6$, C and E, and contain easily absorbed, densely concentrated minerals, especially iron, potassium, magnesium and iodine. Iodine helps to regulate the metabolism by supporting the thyroid in metabolizing fats. Sea vegetables are also high in proteins, carotenes and chlorophyll. Another great attribute of sea vegetables is that they can be added to salads and recipes to lend a "salty" flavor without introducing unhealthy sodium (see page 156), with the added benefit of all the aforementioned nutrients.

When you purchase some sea vegetables, they might come in a hard, dry form. Be sure to rinse them first to wash off any sea salt; then soak them for about ten to fifteen minutes to soften them up. Remember that when rehydrated, dried sea vegetables will expand ten to fifteen times their size. It's a good thing to keep in mind when you are prepping your food!

Best Beauty from the Sea

Arame	Hijiki	Kombu	Wakame
Dulse	Kelp	Nori	

Now that you've met all of the fabulous Beauty Foods, you can see for yourself just how many different delicious, mineral-rich foods you can eat while still cleansing for beauty. You will never feel hungry or unsatisfied on this plan. In fact, the more you clean out the toxic sludge and fuel your body with these nutrient-rich foods, the more satisfied you'll feel!

Now you have the fundamentals of the Beauty Detox Solution. In the next part of this book I'll walk you through some basic detoxing principles and the Beauty Detox phases so that you can put these principles into motion in your life!

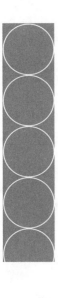

BEAUTY **DETOX** RECAP

○ The mineral- and enzyme-rich Beauty Foods discussed in this chapter are the heart of the program and form the basis of the Beauty Foods Circle—eat them to look and feel your best.

○ Choose plant-based sources of protein and calcium and alkalinizing starches and grains for your Beauty Detox.

○ Fruit is the most life-enhancing food you can eat when your body is alkaline and clean—it's also the strongest cleanser.

○ Enjoy plenty of raw Beauty Greens and Vegetables, and buy organic and local produce whenever possible.

PART TWO

YOUR **BEAUTY** SOLUTION

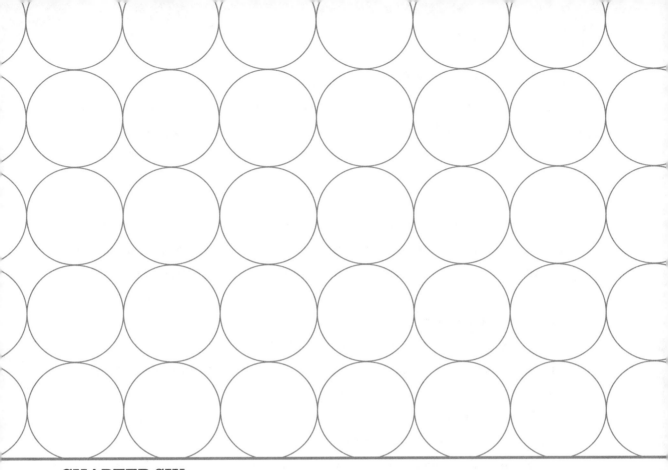

CHAPTER SIX

DETOXING FOR BEAUTY

Except for accidents, all the repair and regeneration of our body must come from within.

—Dr. Norman Walker

Ongoing cleansing is one of the most important ways to reach our highest goals of health and beauty, reverse aging and lose weight. In fact, it might just be *the* most important way. When we hear the word "cleanse," most of us think of it as a noun, as in we do "a cleanse"— usually some kind of fasting or herbal program for a few days here and there, a few times a year. But we actually need to think of cleansing as a *verb* and accelerate and initiate cleans*ing* on an ongoing basis.

During an *Extra* segment I appeared on in February of 2010, Star Jones asked me if I thought cleanses were effective. I replied, "Does it help to clean your house only once or twice a year?" Sure, in many cases doing one cleanse is probably better than doing *nothing*. But can we really get down to the deep garbage and toxicity that have been piling up for years and decades and root them out in only a *few days?* I think not!

Cleansing is how our body rids itself of waste, toxins and the sludge that is trapped inside and is constantly accumulating. Remember our analogy to the clogged wheel? When we are not cleansing properly, we can drive the toxins deeper into our body, where they continue to weaken us, steal our Beauty Energy, make us look old and tired, and eventually cause disease. We as a society are obsessed with putting things *in*, such as the hottest new weight loss pills or herbs, specific mineral supplements and so on. We need to shift our focus to taking things *out.*

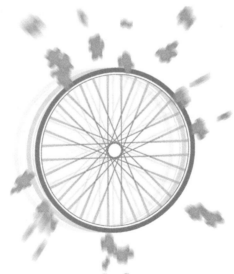

By cleansing, we unclog some of the sludge from our wheel and reverse aging.

We cannot rebuild, heal or maintain our weight easily without cleansing. Cleansing rebalances us and cleans out the sludge and mucus in our bodies so we can adequately absorb nutrients. This is also true for those of us that struggle with being underweight—you will struggle with keeping weight on and getting your body the nutrients it needs until you cleanse out the toxins. If you change your diet but don't cleanse properly on an ongoing basis, you will not get the results you desire, no matter how strictly you adhere to the program.

When you follow the principles outlined in Part 1 of this book, you will begin to kick up toxicity in your system. For this reason it is essential to *cleanse* at the same time. Otherwise, you may feel good for a few months, but if you don't get that newly released toxicity out of the body through these cleansing methods, you will essentially repoison yourself and will feel sick and awful.

The same is true anytime you shift your diet—from omnivore to vegetarian, or vegetarian to vegan, or from vegan to raw foodist. If we don't cleanse properly, the toxicity we kick up through the change in diet will make us feel sick. We then blame it on "not getting enough nutrients" or "being protein deficient," but that is not what is really happening. The reason we are not feeling well is not from a lack in the diet (assuming we are eating the Beauty Detox Solution way, which is a diet packed with whole foods and plant foods!), but because we are being overloaded by newly awakened poisons.

Think of cleansing as reorganizing your entire office. Your files are disorganized and misplaced, every single drawer in your desk is crammed with office supplies and old bills, and there are carefully stacked boxes filled with miscellaneous paperwork. Out of sight, out of mind, right? The week you decide to reorganize your office, at first things look *worse*. You have to take everything out of the drawers and boxes and spread it across the floor to see all the stuff you can *throw away*. No one is denying it can temporarily be somewhat of a painful process and takes some work, and some time. But when you finish, all the boxes are gone, because you got rid of so much junk, and there was enough space in the file cabinets and drawers to put everything away properly! Pounds of garbage have been thrown out, and everything is much, much better. Cleansing the body follows the same principle.

We can also think of detoxification as a similar experience to what a drug addict would experience during withdrawal. When you first take the drug away from the addict, he goes through withdrawal, and symptoms might include fatigue, headaches, diarrhea, constipation, etc. If we give the addict the drug again, he will immediately feel better and his symptoms

⟡ BEAUTY TIP

Cleansing and Looking More Toned

Exercise is important for all of us. I personally love yoga, which teaches us to breathe really deeply and properly, promoting the distribution of oxygen all through the body. Yoga also helps to holistically balance the emotional, mental, spiritual and physical aspects of our being.

When we cleanse, we naturally create more space in our body as waste and trapped gas (generated from fermentation, which can put pressure on our veins and arteries) leave, and there is more room for oxygen to circulate. Oxygen gets more easily to our muscles as our tissues become cleaner.

In my early twenties, I counted each calorie I ate, and I also counted each calorie I burned at the gym on exercise machines. I ran almost every day, and I lifted weights three times a week. Ironically, now I look much more toned across my stomach, arms and legs, even though I have not run or worked out at a gym for years. What a relief! While I still practice yoga and stay active, I don't have to slave away at the gym all the time to look the way I want to. The ongoing cleansing methods I put into practice made, and continue to make, an *enormous* difference. They will be a huge help to you also!

We all need exercise to stay healthy. But we don't have to obsess anymore over excessive exercise routines, because when we put effort into cleansing, we will naturally start to look more toned and lean.

will disappear, as he has *stopped* cleansing. And so it is with us. If we avoid or greatly slow down the detoxification process and its symptoms by going back to eating heavy foods all the time, like pizza, we will stop the ill feelings because we have also stopped cleansing. But we will never really heal! That is why the person on a transition diet who is going through somewhat of a painful detox phase starts to eat chicken again and magically starts to feel better. The discomfort wasn't caused by a protein deficiency, but by loosening up the toxins in the body, and eating the chicken stopped the cleansing process. Don't worry. The cleansing symptoms won't last forever. In fact, most detox symptoms, if they do arise, generally subside within a few weeks.

Toxicity, or sludge, becomes lodged throughout our cells and tissues from years of improper digestion, preservatives in our food and skin-care products, pollution, stress and other factors. We would all be shocked at how much waste is present in the body!

Our eliminative organs, which include the lungs, liver, kidneys, colon and skin, become overwhelmed and are unable to root out all this poison. The body attempts to detoxify in *some* form when its eliminative organs are overwhelmed. These detoxing forms reveal themselves in unwanted acne

The Roots of Western Medicine

Western medicine largely adheres to the doctrines of the French scientist Louis Pasteur, who lived from 1822 to 1895. Pasteur's theories were based on the theory of "germ warfare," which basically hypothesizes that the germs from the outside are what make us sick and create disease. Based on this idea, pretty much all beverages and many foods sold in grocery stores today have been *pasteurized,* or heated to very high temperatures to destroy any potential harmful germs.

But Pasteur had a little-known contemporary and intellectual adversary: fellow French scientist Antoine Beauchamp, who lived from 1816 to 1908. Beauchamp believed the exact opposite. His theory was based on the idea that "the terrain is everything." In other words, it is not just the germs from the outside that cause illness, but a compromised immune system or some predisposing characteristic that allows the germs to flourish in the body and cause illness. For instance, why is it that two people get coughed on directly in the face (gross!) by the same person on the subway, but only one person gets the flu? Dr. Robert Young gives a great analogy to this by pointing out that if you throw seeds on concrete, they cannot grow. But if you throw the seeds on fertile soil, they grow and flourish.[1] And so it is with germs and sickness.

Dr. T. Colin Campbell's findings in *The China Study* support Beauchamp's theories. Campbell discussed how when two experimental groups were exposed to the *same* amount of a carcinogenic substance (such as aflatoxin), the group consuming the higher levels of animal protein and dairy was the one that developed disease (cancer), and the group consuming the lower levels of these foods did not.[2] As Beauchamp theorized, the first group had the right "terrain" for sickness to develop.

Under Beauchamp's theory, we can hypothesize that there really is only *one* disease: an acidic body that releases acidic waste and toxins, compromising immunity. The body then becomes fertile terrain for sickness, disease and harmful bacteria and germs. All the various diseases are symptoms of general toxicity in the body, but not the root cause itself.

This may be why at institutions like the Ann Wigmore Natural Health Institute and the Hippocrates Health Institute, there have been cases where symptoms of diseases such as cancer subside when clients are put on a raw plant diet and cleanse. These institutions do not perform chemotherapy or radiation on specific areas of the body, but rather treat the body holistically and work to raise the alkalinity of the entire body.

Of course, we can see how Pasteur's theory is much more profitable for the pharmaceutical industry, as flu shots, penicillin, other antibiotics and the like make the industry billions of dollars. That is not to say these things don't have an important purpose—clearly they do, and they do save a lot of lives. But if we keep our bodies clean of toxins and excessive waste, balanced at a more alkaline pH and keep our immunity strong, we may need these medicines far less and we ourselves may have much more control over our own health.

or skin eruptions, rashes, colds and flus. So then what? We take medication to suppress the symptoms. The problem is that these drugs do not help with the root cause of the issue—the sludge and toxicity in the body, which have arisen to dangerously high levels. These drugs mask what really needs to happen: cleansing and detoxification.

Here are some typical temporary cleansing symptoms: headaches, sore throat, exhaustion, skin rashes or eruptions, aches and pains, soreness, moodiness, dizziness and light-headedness. You may even temporarily feel a bit more bloated and a few pounds *heavier,* as acidic sludge starts to surface and your body has to hold on to extra water to try to

☙ BEAUTY TIP

Limiting Antibiotics and Other Medications

It used to be that medication and surgery were used primarily for trauma and accidents. In today's world, however, medication is not just readily available, it is very heavily prescribed. In the American culture, we now rely on prescription drugs for pretty much every physical or mental ailment, including sleeping disorders, anxiety, diabetes, depression, heart problems, allergies and acne. And, as Dr. Joel Fuhrman points out in his book *Eat to Live,* these prescription drugs are toxic. He writes, "Doctors learn in their introductory pharmacology course in medical school that all medications are toxic to varying degrees, whether side effects are experienced or not."[3]

Unfortunately, there seem to be a lot of side effects, indeed. An article in *Newsweek* from 1998 entitled "When Drugs Do Harm" explained that "adverse reactions to prescription drugs may rank somewhere between the fourth and sixth leading cause of death in the United States...."[4] Should that surprise us? Medications are manufactured with a cornucopia of chemicals that are toxic to the liver and contribute to acidity, toxemia and overall imbalance in our bodies. They often simply work to just unnaturally suppress the outward symptoms, versus actually correcting the problem itself.

Antibiotics are now casually prescribed for the flu and acne. The major problem with antibiotics is that they kill not only disease-causing bacteria but also our friendly bacteria. As a result, the usually benign yeast *Candida albicans* can multiply, resulting in an overgrowth, which weakens our immune system and disturbs the lining of our intestinal tract.[5] Antibiotics are also commonly fed to factory-farmed animals and get into our body when we consume animal products.

This isn't to say that antibiotics aren't a good thing. Of course there are situations when antibiotics and other medications are lifesavers, but in general we want to reduce and eliminate medications, taking them only when it is absolutely necessary. Our body has incredible power to heal itself if we supply it with the real medicines it needs: a superb diet and ongoing detoxification.

neutralize the waste. These symptoms are usually the strongest in the first few weeks as you shift your diet to the Beauty Detox Solution—if you actually experience them at all. If you stick to the main principles, a large amount of toxins will be flushed out of your body. By the end you will feel and look incredible, and your body will be so much cleaner. Your "office" will have been reorganized.

"Okay, I get that it is important!" you are probably saying. "But how do I actually do it?" Let us get into more specifics. These cleansing methods are crucial to incorporate along with dietary changes to ensure we are eliminating as much toxicity as possible. *Cleansing out toxicity is as important as what we are putting into our bodies.*

BEAUTY DETOX SECRET #1: PROBIOTICS

I wholeheartedly recommend taking a good probiotic every single day. Probiotics help preserve a healthy digestive environment and play a critical role in our immune system, 80 percent of which resides in our gut. As adults we have around four hundred different species and strains of friendly bacteria in our digestive tract. When we are healthy, we should have 80 to 85 percent friendly bacteria. When there is an overbalance of *unfriendly* bacteria in our system, and the percentage of friendly bacteria diminishes, it creates a condition known as dysbiosis.

We talked at length throughout Part 1 about how putrifying, rotting proteins in our intestine create a breeding ground for harmful bacteria and contribute to intestinal toxemia. We can now see that this can be a huge contributing factor to dysbiosis. This imbalance can also be caused by excessive antibiotic consumption (both directly and from consuming meat and dairy products containing antibiotics), consuming too many artificial chemicals and sugar, taking medications, drinking chlorinated and fluorinated water, poor digestion and constipation, and living in our stressful and pollution-filled world in general!

Probiotics can help restore our internal balance and will increase our vibrancy and overall health in the following ways:

- Improve digestive functions, helping to eliminate constipation and diarrhea
- Improve liver function
- Improve resistance to allergies
- Improve vitamin synthesis, and specifically the manufacturing of B vitamins

- ○ Increase energy
- ○ Improve the absorption of nutrients
- ○ Help eliminate bloating and heartburn

◝ BEAUTY TIP

How Our Face Reveals Inner Health

For over five thousand years in Chinese medicine, practitioners have understood that uneven color and texture, patchiness, lines, breakouts, and other issues with our face are really indicative of deeper issues going on within our bodies and in our organs.[6] Here are some commonly held ancient Chinese beliefs about what we might learn from examining our face:

Breakouts around the chin/jaw area could indicate a hormonal imbalance and congestion in the colon.

Lines above the upper lip might indicate stagnation or blockages in the digestive tract, specifically relating to the organs of the stomach and small intestines. This can be attributed to the accumulation of acidic waste and toxicity, which is not adequately leaving the body.

Deep laugh lines (and the nasolabial line) relate to our lung line and liver. These lines could be due to smoking or shallow chest breathing, so that not enough oxygen is getting into the lungs (yoga definitely helps with this!), or a colon that is so backed up that our lung meridian is being impeded. It can also indicate an overloaded liver.

A lined forehead might point to congestion, and specifically a blocked, toxin-filled colon and gallbladder. Big contributors to this can be consuming a lot of dairy, cooked oils or processed foods. On the other hand, one might have a good diet but is not cleansing properly or adequately to keep up with the toxicity the good diet is kicking up.

Dark under-eye circles or puffiness can indicate adrenal exhaustion. Too much caffeine, a lack of sleep and too much stress can cause this.

Crow's-feet around the eyes can also indicate that our adrenals are being overtaxed and that our bodies are acidic and imbalanced.

Patchy skin or lines high up around the cheekbone area may be associated with heart issues. Eating too much clogging animal protein, too many animal products, or cooked oil could be a major contributor.

The good news is that our cells regenerate. If we take positive steps now to improve our diet and cleanse our bodies, we can reverse issues and make major improvements in our overall heath and beauty!

When it comes to choosing a probiotic supplement, keep in mind that there are numerous probiotics available in the marketplace. However, many of them aren't as effective as they could or should be. Probiotics are living organisms, and like other living organisms they are susceptible to death. The benefits of probiotics are realized only when the *live* probiotic cells make their way to the intestine. The harsh environment of the human stomach kills a good portion of the live cells before they can reach the intestine and benefit our health. When shopping for a probiotic, be sure to look for one that has a specialized delivery system designed to support the safe transport of live cells into the intestine. Also, it is important that there is not just a high culture count overall, but that there is a high culture count of a variety of highly beneficial strains. *Lactobacillus acidophilus* is a common strain and is particularly useful to get candida under control. *Bifidobacterium bifidum* assists with promoting general immunity.

BEAUTY DETOX SECRET #2: PLANT-BASED DIGESTIVE ENZYMES

We've already discussed how important enzymes are to our health and beauty. Over the years, our enzyme reserve becomes diminished. Therefore, our body may not be digesting foods, even properly combined foods, as well as it once did when we were children. We know now that any amount of poorly digested food ferments and putrefies in the digestive tract, stimulating the growth of unfriendly bacteria and the creation of their toxic, acidic by-products and waste, which then become absorbed into the blood and deposited in tissues all around the body, especially soft-tissue areas, such as the joints.[7] Toxins in the blood also negatively affect our skin and our physical appearance!

Digestive enzymes are therefore a critical aid to us. They can be taken daily and right before meals and should be ingested before any meal that contains cooked food. They give our bodies an extra boost of lipase, amylase and protease, to help efficiently digest fats, starches and proteins. We could *all* use the boost!

Here are some of their specific benefits:

○ Improve the absorption and assimilation of Beauty Minerals and nutrients
○ Help to slow the aging process by preserving the body's own enzymes
○ Promote efficient digestion

○ Free up Beauty Energy to rebuild and replace damaged cells, including the collagen of the skin

○ Increase energy

○ Enhance cleansing, which can improve acne and other imbalances

○ Decrease bloating, gassiness and constipation

When you choose a digestive enzyme supplement, be sure to look for one that is vegan and plant-based, rather than one that contains enzymes from bovine animals (cows or oxen) or other animals or animal products. Plant enzymes may be more active at a fuller pH range than animal-based enzymes. Choose a supplement that contains a blend of lipase, amylase and protease, to help efficiently digest fats, starches and proteins. Cellulase is another category of digestive enzymes and can also be useful in a supplement, as it breaks down cellulose and chitin, a fiber similar to cellulose that is found in the cell wall of candida.[8]

BEAUTY DETOX SECRET #3: PROBIOTIC & ENZYME SALAD

Probiotic & Enzyme Salad is composed of raw, cultured vegetables that have been chopped and left in airtight glass containers at room temperature for several days. This allows the

🍃 BEAUTY TIP

The Power of Raw Apple Cider Vinegar

Raw apple cider vinegar is the only acceptable vinegar we want to consume on a regular basis, since it is non-acid-forming. I know… you are probably wondering what will become of one of your favorite salad dressing ingredients—balsamic vinegar. Balsamic vinegar is okay for special occasions, like weddings and formal sit-down dinners, where the salads are always pre-made. But since it is so acid-forming, it should *not* be an everyday staple in our diet.

More about the good stuff! Raw apple cider vinegar actually helps promote optimal digestion and encourages the growth of friendly bacteria in our bodies. It is great in salad dressings. An age-old digestive remedy calls for sipping one tablespoon of the vinegar diluted in a cup of water twenty minutes before meals. Raw apple cider vinegar is high in minerals and potassium, which help promote cellular cleansing. It has antiseptic qualities and can help cleanse our digestive tract, and it promotes bowel movements.

Be sure that you buy a brand labeled "raw" and "unfiltered." Pasteurized apple cider vinegar does not have these healing properties!

beneficial lactobacilli and enzymes that are already naturally present in the vegetables to flourish, creating a food that is extremely rich in probiotics (friendly bacteria), enzymes and minerals. It is really raw sauerkraut, but usually when we hear that word, we think of the soggy, salty food that is sold at hot dog stands or in supermarkets to add to meat products. That is not what we are talking about here! Commercial sauerkraut is loaded with refined salt and pasteurized to high temperatures, which destroys its important benefits. Raw sauerkraut is a powerful source of probiotics and enzymes—two essentials for healthy digestion, improved Beauty Energy and ongoing cleansing.

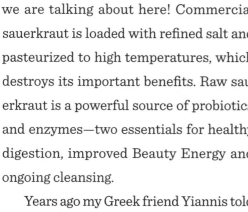

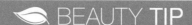 BEAUTY TIP

Yogurt and Kefir

Many people look to yogurt and kefir as sources of probiotics. I do not recommend consuming yogurt, which is made of pasteurized dairy milk. Pasteurized dairy products are clogging foods and contain high levels of the protein casein. Having yogurt in the morning, when most of us want to eat it, is especially clogging as it creates a traffic jam right in the beginning of our whole day. There really is no purpose for yogurt when we are taking a daily probiotic and regularly eating Probiotic & Enzyme Salad. If you can find raw goat's milk kefir (which may be difficult to get a hold of), that would be an acceptable choice and easier to digest than any cow's milk products, though it is certainly not recommended as a daily food.

Years ago my Greek friend Yiannis told me about a farm with a table at the Union Square farmers' market that sold delicious raw sauerkraut and other cultured vegetables. Since I frequent that farmers' market several times a week, I decided to check it out. I had studied the benefits of cultured foods and had tried some of Dr. Ann Wigmore's rejuvelac recipe, but I had really never consumed cultured foods regularly to experience the benefits firsthand.

I loved the taste, and I began to pile raw sauerkraut on my daily dinner salads and sometimes had it at lunch. I also found that if I happened to be eating grains, like millet, or a protein dish, like a nut pâté, the raw sauerkraut greatly helped me digest the other foods. I had more energy and, yes, I was going to the bathroom much more frequently. Exciting stuff!

I am now convinced that raw, cultured vegetables are among the most important foods of our modern day. As they are powerful, extremely helpful weapons to clean out sludge, and to look younger and more radiant, I like calling these powerful raw, cultured veggies Probiotic & Enzyme Salad, so we are reminded of their key benefits.

While cultured foods are a critical food group in many cultures, such as kimchi in Korea and kefir in Russia, the American diet and the Western diet in general are sorely lacking in these foods. Moreover, any amount of friendly bacteria that may be present in our food supply is destroyed by the commercial food industry. Our produce is sprayed with chemicals and contaminants and grown in soil stripped of beneficial microorganisms, and livestock and other animals are often fed with grains that have been chemically altered and laced with antibiotics and steroids.

Because of this, we need to make the effort to seek out and consume these cultured foods, which help repopulate our intestinal tracts!

BEAUTY BENEFITS OF PROBIOTIC & ENZYME SALAD:

o **Frees up Beauty Energy.** Raw, cultured veggies are teaming with potent friendly bacteria and enzymes. Probiotic & Enzyme Salad helps digest other foods that are eaten with it, freeing up Beauty Energy. This is very important to note for our weight loss goals! If we eat Probiotic & Enzyme Salad alongside both starches and proteins, including miscombined Beauty Food Pairings, it helps everything digest much better.

o **Increases our Beauty Enzyme reserve.** The friendly bacteria are packed with enzymes, so they help maintain our body's enzyme reserves. The more enzymes we have, the more our bodies have energy to rebuild our skin, our hair, and help us lose excess weight.

o **Helps eliminate toxins and speeds cleansing.** The raw, cultured vegetables in our Probiotic & Enzyme Salad are such powerful detoxifiers that when we consume them, they immediately start rebalancing our intestine. They attack toxic sludge and loosen hard and encrusted fecal matter. Okay, while the image is grotesque, that is great news! During this process, we might experience more gas and bloating as we detox and the sludge becomes unlodged. This is only a temporary stage and will pass. To ease the discomfort of excessive gas, a colonic or enema might be very helpful.

o **Restores the balance of friendly bacteria in the body.** The natural probiotics help replenish the good flora in our digestive tract.

o **Helps control sugar cravings and reduces appetite.** Probiotic & Enzyme Salad helps us feel full and reduces our cravings for sweets. This is extremely helpful as we work to cut soda, ice cream, cookies, bread, pasta, dairy, doughnuts, and otherrefined sugars and carbohydrates out of our diet.

As our inner balance of good bacteria is restored in the body, we're better able to shed excess weight and our skin improves. Our energy will become more vibrant. Because these functions are so important, we must consume Probiotic & Enzyme Salad regularly in addition to taking a probiotic supplement and digestive enzymes. You may wonder, *Why can't we just pop the pills and that's enough?* For the best results, we must *also* consume food sources for maximum absorption and assimilation, that is, to bring larger quantities of beneficial nutrients into our bodies.

While we can buy raw, cultured veggies in health food stores (look for jars of raw sauerkraut in the refrigerated section—but avoid the brands that contain excessive salt), they are very easy and inexpensive to prepare in large batches at home, to ensure you can enjoy them regularly. All it takes is a little bit of time to chop and store! Trust me when I say it is really easy. And it is completely worth it for the benefits that come with regularly consuming these veggies. As we shift our diet and want to greatly improve how we look and how we feel, regularly eating Probiotic & Enzyme Salad is extremely important. Consuming one half to one cup with dinner at least five nights a week would be ideal. Check out the recipe for Probiotic & Enzyme Salad in Chapter 11. With some planning, we should have these foods available to us in our own refrigerators for the cost of a few cents a day.

BEAUTY DETOX SECRET #4: MAGNESIUM-OXYGEN SUPPLEMENT

This powerful cleanser combines magnesium oxide compounds that have been ozonated and stabilized to release monatomic, or nascent, oxygen over twelve hours or more throughout the entire digestive system. The magnesium acts as a vehicle to transport the oxygen throughout the body and has the gentle effect of loosening toxins and acidic waste and transporting them out of the body.

Oxygen also supports the growth of friendly bacteria, which is essential for proper digestive and intestinal health. Magnesium-oxygen supplements are safe for regular use and provide daily ongoing detoxification. Be sure to follow the directions on the label, and simply reduce the dosage or take the supplement less frequently if you experience any adverse reactions.

Here are some of a magnesium-oxygen supplement's specific benefits:

○ Increases oxygenation in the body, which has a remarkable cleansing effect without being an irritant

○ Breaks down, detoxifies and eliminates impacted toxic waste material that has accumulated in the digestive tract

○ May help to balance pH in the body as it works to clean out old, acidic waste

○ Enhances the body's cleansing functions, which can assist with acne and other imbalances

○ Decreases bloating, gassiness and constipation

Unlike synthetic laxatives, or even harsh natural herbs with laxative properties, like senna, good-quality magnesium-oxygen supplements are non-habit-forming and promote the strength of all the organs' functions, making them safe for regular use.

This supplement has been a huge help in my personal journey to continue cleansing myself, and I have tried many different brands, as well as powders (yuck!) and capsules. It has been indispensible for my clients who do not have access to colonics, can't afford them or simply refuse to get them. For your Beauty Detox, it is absolutely critical to consistently pull sludge out of your wheel, in addition to eating the right foods! This supplement is designed to help us do just that.

BEAUTY DETOX SECRET #5: GRAVITY-CENTERED COLONICS AND ENEMAS

Colonics are a professional procedure that cost about $50 to $125. While they are somewhat pricey, I firmly believe that properly administered colonics are one of the greatest cleansing methods there is. In this type of colonic, water is administered into the rectum by a speculum with split tubing, which simultaneously allows clean water to flow into the colon while waste flows out of the body and directly into the sewage.

Okay, I know it doesn't sound like *fun* per se. But having a colonic is like having the underside of your car power washed for forty-five minutes. The gravity-method colonic shouldn't hurt or feel excessively uncomfortable. The gentle pressure of warm water helps dissolve old waste from the walls of your colon and takes it right out. This old sludge in our digestive tract must be removed to help keep our "wheels" clear! Even if we go to the

True Beauty Story

ANTONIA GIOVANNI IS A WARM, BUBBLY ITALIAN WOMAN IN HER EARLY FIFTIES. She loves to spoil her large family with her homemade cooking, which is usually pretty elaborate and involves different courses. Actually, it was her twenty-five-year-old daughter that contacted me. She was worried about her mother, Antonia, because she was over fifty pounds overweight—a lot for Antonia's five-foot frame. Her mother was already on blood pressure medication and no longer had the energy she once had to do her own food shopping and run errands. She was spending more and more time in front of the television or perched on the stoop of her Brooklyn home, talking to neighbors that came by to see her.

When I met Antonia, she *immediately* made it clear to me that being a vegetarian was not an option. I assured her that she didn't have to become one. We took a look at her diet and started making adjustments, especially early on in the day. We added a lot more raw vegetables and lightened her lunch meals.

Dinnertime was the highlight of her day, and there were frequent occurrences of improper Beauty Pairings (meatballs and pasta, breaded chicken!). However, I knew that with Antonia's cultural upbringing and love of making elaborate dinners for her family, we could not cut all of that out. At least not all at once. We made a deal: she could keep some of what she was eating if she reduced her portions and started adding the Probiotic & Enzyme Salad to all her dinner meals.

Making the Probiotic & Enzyme Salad at home was so easy for her, especially since she was an Italian chef. She thought it was "no big deal." And she didn't mind the taste at all. Well, it *was* a big deal when it came to her health! With the dietary changes we made, she started losing weight within a few weeks. The Probiotic & Enzyme Salad was making her so full that her portion sizes for the other foods were even smaller than what we had talked about. Plus, what she was eating was digesting so much better! She was usually too full for dessert and had lost much of her taste for it.

She was going to the bathroom much more, her energy was higher, and after five months she had already lost over twenty-eight pounds. We still have a lot of work to do, but we are on the way! The Probiotic & Enzyme Salad has been key to not only reducing her appetite but also to attacking and rooting out the old sludge to rebalance her internally.

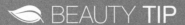

BEAUTY TIP

Senna

There are some herbs on the market today, such as senna and cascara, that have been promoted by certain short-term cleanse programs as laxatives. These herbs are only okay *very occasionally*, such as when we are very constipated from a day or two of traveling. But when taken regularly, these herbs can actually weaken our adrenals. Weak adrenals and reduced energy in the long term are actually a contributing factor to constipation. Senna should *not* be consumed habitually.

bathroom a lot, most of us would be *shocked* at how much waste our body can and does hold in our colon, which has the ability to expand and store increasing amounts of garbage. Remember, our bodies are a hot 98.6 degrees, and all that stuck toxic waste can really bake in there!

Our colon is the sewer system of the body and encases a large amount of the aging sludge we have been talking about. When our colon becomes overloaded, toxicity builds in the rest of our digestive tract, including our liver, kidneys, etc. When we clean the colon, we start a chain reaction of cleansing in other organs throughout the whole body.

Though it may sound counterintuitive, the more our diet improves, the more often we should get colonics. As we cleanse and wake up toxicity, colonics help remove the massive amounts of waste that have been hidden in our bodies. Colonics are excellent aids for helping with acne and skin eruptions, as well. *But if we don't change our diet first, colonics won't work very well.*

Check out your local area for gravity-centered practitioners. Gravity-centered colonics typically do not cause major discomfort from having to "hold" water in the body, an issue

BEAUTY TIP

Bring Color Back to Gray Hair

Gray hair can be an indication that our bodies are not properly absorbing proteins and minerals. As we clean out our digestive tract and improve our diet to include more mineral- and enzyme-rich foods, we might very well see our hair return to its original color! The great Dr. Ann Wigmore, who advocated eating a large percentage of raw greens and blended raw green drinks, and having colonics, had her gray hair turn back to jet-black naturally!

usually associated with hydraulic pressure colonics. Some people think colonics are "bad" because they can wash out some friendly bacteria from your digestive tract. But we can rest assured that any friendly bacteria that might be removed are easily replaced with a daily probiotic supplement and the consumption of Probiotic & Enzyme Salad. Gravity-centered colonics also work with gravity and your body's energy to release waste, so you'll actually strengthen peristalsis and your body's natural bowel moments, not weaken them.

ENEMAS: THE ALTERNATIVE TO A COLONIC

There really is no substitute for getting a gravity-centered colonic, but it is not always convenient or affordable for everyone. In these cases, another option would be an enema kit, which you can self-administer. You can get enema kits at certain drugstores. With an enema, you release fresh water into the rectum through a tube connected to a bag as you lie relaxing on your side and then sit on the toilet to release old matter. Do this multiple times. Be sure to follow the instructions that come with the enema kit closely. If you are releasing only dirty water and no actual waste, then you should stop the process, as you may be backing yourself up more, and try it again a few days later.

Remember, a cleansed body is one that can regenerate, heal and take in fresh nutrients. How we are cleaning out the sludge is just as important as improving the quality, combination and order of foods we are putting into our body. It is our key to growing younger and more beautiful and becoming more vibrant!

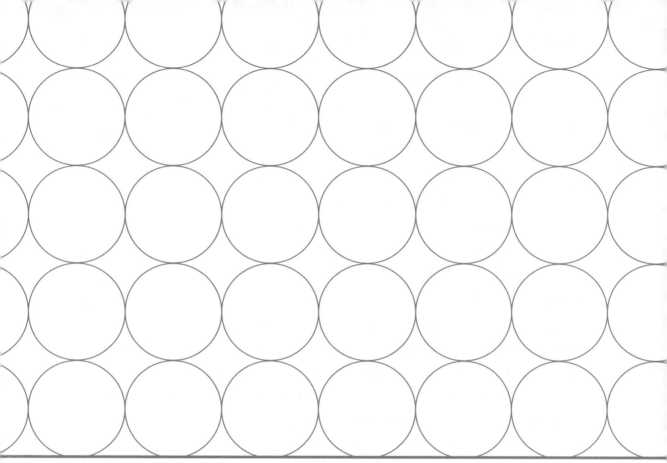

CHAPTER SEVEN

BECOMING BEAUTIFUL

The world will be saved by beauty.

—Fyodor Dostoyevsky
The Brothers Karamazov

In the next few chapters I'll walk you through the three-phase Beauty Detox program. These pages hold the key to putting the powerful cleansing practices I talk about throughout the book into practice. Before too long, you'll start to see the results with clearer skin, reduced eye circles, shinier hair and a healthy, radiant glow. And from the very start you'll experience the results in terms of renewed energy that stays strong through the day and diminished stress—you will actually feel the difference when you free up Beauty Energy!

Before we dive in, it's crucial to understand how important it is to pace yourself throughout this process. When we begin to see how we can directly affect our health and beauty with alkalinity, it is easy to get really enthusiastic and want to do a complete overhaul of our diet or jump to the conclusion that we should eat only raw fruits and vegetables...starting right now! That's what happened to me. I was so fascinated with the concepts I was learning that I made drastic changes overnight. I didn't suffer any severe trauma, but I did hit physical and mental roadblocks and detox walls along the way, which I want to help you avoid.

Moreover, I now believe that eating all raw food or trying to stick to any dietary classification (raw foodist, etc.) is not always realistic, nor is it necessarily compatible with everyone's genetic makeup or lifestyle. Plus, incorporating the right kind of cooked food that digests easily can be highly beneficial and helps keep us on the overall plan. I personally do eat some cooked food (veggies and alkaline grains) now and feel better than ever! A diet with a lot of alkaline foods and some cooked foods is more healthy than the diet of raw foodists who eat a ton of agave, dehydrated, concentrated foods and copious amounts of oil!

THE IMPORTANCE OF TRANSITIONING

Transitioning the diet is key to the Beauty Detox Solution. We already discussed this a bit in the Ongoing Cleansing section, but it is so important, it is worth mentioning again. Most people never talk about transitioning, but it is one of the vital keys to long-term success. Why? Well, consider that most of us have spent at least a few *decades* eating acidic foods, the putrefying and fermenting residue of which is lodged as sludge, in varying degrees, in different parts of our body. If we decide one day to make a radical shift to a diet with a high percentage of alkaline foods, namely fruits and vegetables, we are also unleashing the strongest possible cleansers that we can put into our bodies.

What happens when we pour a dozen bottles of Drano down a clogged pipe? We peel free a massive amount of matter from the sides of the pipe, and we better be sure that this old matter leaves the pipe altogether. Otherwise it will get stuck right in the middle and we will be worse off than if we had just left it all encrusted on the sides of the pipe!

This is exactly what can happen when we make drastic switches in our diet very quickly, even when we are incorporating very good foods. We wake up sleeping demons that are in the form of toxic waste! If we neglect to wake up a *limited* amount of toxins at a time, which can then leave the body in a controlled way, we might experience very unpleasant side effects, such as headaches, nausea, dizziness, breakouts and other skin eruptions, and diarrhea, and actually feel quite sick. In some cases, as lots of acidic waste is kicked up, our body has to retain more water to neutralize it, and we might feel a couple of pounds heavier right in the beginning. Don't worry. This will go away!

It is essential to transition our diet properly. If the toxins don't leave the body quickly, or don't all leave, all we've done is reawaken poison and bring it to the surface, where it will be reabsorbed by the tissues. I've seen it way too many times with overly enthusiastic clients and readers of my blog! Oftentimes when people make a transition to more alkaline foods and become vegetarians, they feel weak. Their friends and family say, "See? You can't eat that way. It doesn't suit your body, and you are deficient in protein and nutrients!" Have you ever met someone who tried to become a vegetarian and started to feel awful after a few weeks or months? That person goes back to eating meat and how he or she was eating before and immediately starts feeling *better.* Why?

What is actually happening is *not* a lack of nutrition in the body or a lack of some key nutrient, like protein (assuming that person is eating the greens and plant food–based Beauty Detox way). Rather, that person is getting poisoned from the inside out by toxins, which the newly integrated, powerfully cleansing foods have shaken loose. Those very poisons are the acidic, toxic residue that keeps us from efficiently absorbing nutrients into our body. That is why transitioning and cleansing along the way are so crucial to break through to new levels of health, healing and beauty.

The three phases of the Beauty Detox Solution—Blossoming Beauty, Radiant Beauty and True Beauty—take this into account. Transitioning your detox from phase to phase so that you arrive at a diet with a high percentage of alkaline foods over time and in a controlled manner is critical. No matter which phase you are in, you will see results.

The Beauty Detox Solution is not a "cleanse" or "diet" in the sense that it is something that we adopt for twenty-one days or a few months, only to go back to our old ways. It truly is a long-term way of eating. It is a lifestyle, and therefore there is no need to "sprint" and get there immediately. Take your time making changes along the way, and definitely slow down your transition while still applying the broad principles and paradigm of whichever phase you are in.

True Beauty Story

SARAH LEWIS, AGE TWENTY-FIVE, IS A CLASSIC EXAMPLE OF SOMEONE PROCEEDING too quickly with dietary changes. She is a reader from Denver, Colorado, who found my blog and we started doing phone consultations. Her main goals were to drop about seven pounds and improve her skin. We talked about making gradual changes so her body could catch up and she would not detox too quickly. She started making some changes, and she dropped three pounds in the first week and a half. Her energy became really high and, instead of taking the gradual steps we talked about, she got so excited that she went from a partially cooked, meat-filled diet to raw food veganism within a mere few weeks.

I got a call from her one afternoon, and her voice sounded hollow and far away. I thought we had a bad connection. But then she piped up. "I'm on the floor of my bathroom. I'm really light-headed, and I have diarrhea and a bad headache. I don't feel great." Sarah had suddenly gone from feeling like a million bucks to feeling at a very low point. She had made changes too quickly, and her diet had awoken toxins that her body was struggling to eliminate. I counseled her, saying, "It's not that you are deficient in anything. It is not that this diet doesn't work for you. It is that you have changed your diet too quickly without cleansing!"

We brought in cooked and heavier foods to slow down the cleansing process, then adopted a reasonable transition level. She felt better quickly and learned her lesson! Now it has been over fourteen months since we started working together. She has made many great shifts in her diet, though she decided that being a 100 percent raw vegan is not for her. Nor does she need to be. She enjoys fish, eggs and healthy grains. She has lost ten pounds, her skin looks great, and her body has firmed up. She sent me a recent picture and she looks gorgeous! We have found a balanced diet that is right for her, one that makes her feel great and that suits her lifestyle.

THE BEAUTY PHASES

This is *your* time. You can do this. Make it your own and own it! There is a phase to fit your lifestyle, budget and where you are right now.

FIND YOUR BEAUTY PHASE

Now the real excitement can begin! Now that you have read all of Part 1 (and you have, haven't you?), you have a firm understanding of why the phases are structured as they are. You have new insight into evaluating which foods are healthy and why, and you have learned new information on how to properly combine your foods and order them throughout the day to maximize Beauty Energy.

Regardless of which phase you enter into, you will experience huge improvements as your body takes in a tremendous amount of alkaline-forming, chlorophyll-rich plant foods, and true antiaging can begin as we start to unearth the sludge. Though this may be a totally different way of eating than you are used to, or may go against some information you heard in the past, I am confident that once you start to experience the results for yourself, you'll know that you truly have found the Beauty Detox Solution!

BLOSSOMING BEAUTY

In this phase you have adequate time to adjust to your new, alkaline-forming diet, made up primarily of foods from the Beauty Food Circle. Not only do you not have to buy any new kitchen equipment, but many of the foods are upgraded variations of foods with which you are already familiar. Even without making drastic changes to your diet, you will still make huge progress thanks to all the alkalizing greens and proper food combinations you'll be enjoying! You will have more energy and less bloat, and you will lose weight, especially in the belly area.

In order to avoid making changes too quickly, you will consume some cooked grains for breakfast and lunch. Animal products can be kept in your diet, except for dairy, but you will cut them out of lunch, since they can disrupt your Light to Heavy food order, and should be consumed only once per day at a maximum. You'll cut out highly refined sugars and carbs, and start to wean yourself off of gluten-containing foods, like wheat, rye and barley, which cause bloating and are difficult to digest. But you won't miss any of those foods, anyway, as we have Beauty Grains, such as quinoa and millet, and products made of them, such as bread, crackers and pasta.

If you are more than fifty pounds overweight, are exhausted, suspect you have candida, have a lot of skin issues and/or are an absolute beginner, I recommend starting with Blossoming Beauty. If these concepts seem totally foreign to you and you are used to eating some form of animal protein five times a day, Blossoming Beauty may be the right place to start. If you are keen to start on the Glowing Green Smoothie and don't have any of the aforementioned issues, you might just try diving into Radiant Beauty!

RADIANT BEAUTY

In this phase you start enjoying the Glowing Green Smoothie, which is super exciting! You will eat only alkaline-forming plant foods in the mornings—no more cooked grains for breakfast. This extends the "cleanse mode" that your body has been in through the whole night, so that the hours that you are cleansing start to add up on a daily and weekly basis, and you are consistently getting more sludge out of your wheel!

You'll reduce your intake of animal products further, but you can still have them a few times a week, especially fish and eggs. You will have lots of beautifying fats from avocados, as well as all the Beauty Grains and the products that come from them.

This is the phase where you may experience the biggest results and lose the most weight! Your skin will start to glow and become smooth, your under-eye circles will diminish and your hair will start to shine.

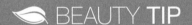 BEAUTY TIP

Stick to It!

We are all improving as long as we don't give up! Stick to the phase you are in, and if you stray, get right back on the path. You *do* have the inner strength and power to improve your health and look gorgeous. Keep your bigger goals in mind. Visualize how you want to look and feel, and stick to that clear picture. This is your time! Make it yours. Own it.

TRUE BEAUTY

In this phase you drink the Glowing Green Juice in the morning (or stick with the fiber-containing Glowing Green Smoothie if you like). You'll reduce the amount of animal products in you diet to only a small portion of fish, eggs and goat's cheese, eliminating land animals altogether. Once you get to this point in the program, you may decide that you don't want to eat any animal products at all.

You'll eliminate cooked grains not only in the mornings but also at lunch and in the middle of the day, which keeps the "road" even more clear and accelerates cleansing for longer periods of time.

This is a pretty high level of diet that may not work for everyone's lifestyle or genetic makeup. If you moved to this phase from Radiant Beauty but simply find it to be a daily struggle and too much effort, or feel too deprived or too obsessive about your diet, then you should move back down to the Radiant Beauty phase. That might just be the right phase for you over the long term! But if the True Beauty phase feels right to you, you will be rewarded with a very high level of health and beauty.

GENERAL GUIDELINES FOR TRANSITIONING

- Stay in each phase at least one month before moving on.

- If you are feeling good in a certain phase, you can stay there for as long as you want. You will improve at any level, though you will see the most radical change when you progress to (or begin at) Radiant Beauty and start enjoying the Glowing Green Smoothie. When you want to achieve higher results, you can move forward and try the next phase. The degree to which you want to improve, and the current state of your health, will dictate how quickly you move up to a different phase.

- If you *are* losing weight and feeling good, but it requires debilitating discipline—you are constantly dreaming of food and your will is keeping you on the path, but part of you wants to eat the way you used to—you are not ready to move up yet! Cravings mean that your body is still finding the diet too restrictive. Drop down to the next level or stay where you are for as long as it feels comfortable and natural. Stay in a phase until the lifestyle feels automatic, that is, until you don't have to think about it, as it has become ingrained in your life. If you move up before then, you will feel deprived and will "cheat."

- Avoid feeling judgmental and competitive with yourself, or attacking yourself for feeling weak at times. Remember we are creating a whole new lifestyle that is meant to last the rest of your life. Take your time transitioning!

- The best idea is to keep things simple. What we need more than anything is salads and lots of greens. We have to retrain ourselves to regard salad as the *main* part of our meal, not an appetizer or a side dish. Instead of fancy recipes, focus on creating a few basic salads and vegetable/grain dishes that you love and that can be your staples.

What about Salt?

Many of us might have liberally sprinkled salt on our foods in the past. It is, after all, usually readily available on the tables of nearly every single restaurant, as well as perhaps our own kitchen table.

We might also have reasoned that salt is a condiment that has no calories but still has the power to transform bland foods into tasty treats. Well, those days of unbridled salt consumption are over! We are striving to achieve excellent health and beauty. Too much salt, and especially the wrong kind of salt, can seriously set us back in those goals. Salt can contribute to increasing the risk for heart disease, hypertension, high blood pressure and kidney disease.

There is absolutely no moderation involved when it comes to table salt, which is really denatured sodium chloride. It is poison in our bodies and we must expel it *completely* from out diet starting today. It is a "hungry," or biologically incomplete, molecule that leaches calcium and other minerals out of our body in our urine when an excess is excreted. Table salt is dead, kiln-dried, highly processed and highly toxic, and thus it poses a threat to the health of your body. Table salt also creates "false fat," making us look bloated and pounds heavier than we truly are. We must avoid it at all cost. Throw it out of your cabinet right now! Resist the urge to add any to your food from saltshakers wherever you are.

With careful moderation, we may use high-quality sea salt, such as Celtic sea salt or Himalayan sea salt, in certain recipes. These sea salts have been dried by the sun and wind, so they are raw and contain enzymes and around seventy trace minerals and trace elements. They include the mineral magnesium, which is involved in over three hundred detoxification pathways in the body and is present in sea salt only when it contains moisture. (Check the label to be sure it says "dried by the sun and wind.") Cheaper varieties of sea salt can still be kiln-dried under high heat.

Sea vegetables, such as dulse, have a salty taste but are low in sodium and are great to add to salads and veggie dishes instead of salt. The less straight salt we use, the better. A thousand to fifteen hundred milligrams of sodium per day *or less* is a good daily quota. Most of us are used to a very salty flavor because we consume so many processed foods, which have lots of salt. As we move away from these processed foods and toward natural foods, our ability to detect and appreciate subtle flavors will increase and we won't miss adding all that excessive salt to our food at all!

BEAUTY PHASE PRINCIPLES

Following is the crux of the program—the core principles to follow for *each* beauty phase.

1 | **Remember Your Beauty Foods.**

Remember that the whole plan is based on a diet made up largely of raw plant foods. These are our real food heroes. They provide the minerals, vitamins, amino acids, fiber and other nutrients that we need to feel and look our best.

Here are some key reminders:

○ Raw plant foods should be the majority of the meal and should always go in the body first. The salad, which comes first, is not merely an appetizer, but the biggest and bulkiest part of the meal. Remember the Beauty Food Circle, and try to stick to 80 percent alkaline-forming foods at each meal (if not more).

○ In Phase 2 the green drinks start coming into play. Resist the urge to chug them! Make a chewing action as you drink them so they can mix thoroughly with saliva to get the digestive process going and maximize nutrients. If you drink them too fast, you might get bloated, which we definitely want to avoid.

○ Be prepared! If you are going to a party, traveling, eating out at a Chinese restaurant, or encounter any other situation where you know raw vegetables might be hard to come by, keep some carrots or celery on hand to eat an hour beforehand.

○ Refined carbs in the form of refined, processed starch and processed or artificial sugars are completely off the menu. Refer to Chapter 5 for more Beauty Grains and Starches.

○ Dairy is not beautiful and is avoided in all the phases. If you need a few reminders of why, please refer to the dairy section in Chapter 5, on page 99.

What about Supplements?

Supplements should *never* be deemed a substitute for a healthy diet packed with fresh greens and other produce. However, I often recommend to my clients that they take a high-quality, whole-food-based and nonsynthetic multivitamin/multimineral supplement if they are worried that they aren't eating perfectly. It can be good insurance. Most all of us need to supplement with vitamin D_3, and my vegan friends should supplement with B_{12}. Other than that, be sure to pick up a probiotic supplement, digestive enzymes, a magnesium-oxygen supplement and ground or fresh flaxseeds (one tablespoon of the flaxseeds have daily omega-3 fats).

2 | **Eat Only When You Are Hungry.**
Never eat when you are not hungry, such as when you first wake up in the morning. Resist eating just "because it is breakfast time." Wait until you genuinely need food. Over time, as our bodies become healthy and balanced, we will be much more in touch with our true hunger.

3 | **Follow Beauty Food Pairing and Eat Light to Heavy.**
It is imperative that we pay attention to the order and combination of foods we are eating, that is, to our Beauty Pairing Principle and our Light to Heavy Principle, as this is key to making progress and key to the whole program. The order and combination keep food moving through our body, and these principles should never be broken, except for the occasional dinner mishap.

During the day, we feast on plant food, which includes green drinks, water- and fiber-filled salads, veggies and fruit. Plant food makes us more beautiful the more we eat it! Dinner is the only meal when we will consume concentrated proteins, so we don't cause a traffic jam and are able to free up Beauty Energy for as long as possible during the day.

BEAUTY TIP

Eating Out

It is totally possible (and easy!) to eat in restaurants while staying on this plan, whatever phase you are in. You will not be required to order or eat weird or difficult-to-find foods. You'll see that there is enough variety in the plan to be able to stick to it, eat in most restaurants and enjoy different cuisines. Always start with a salad. If a restaurant has really wimpy little side salads, you might want to get a double order, as I often do. Make a choice as to whether you are going to have a concentrated *starch* or a concentrated *protein* meal, along with vegetables, and order around the choice you made. For instance, you could order salad, followed by fish and veggies, *or* salad followed by pasta with marinara sauce or brown rice and veggies.

Asian restaurants, especially Thai, are among the easiest restaurants to eat out at because there are so many vegetable entrées you can order. I always try to steer family, friends or business associates in that direction. If you are going to a nice Italian restaurant and love pizza, they can probably make it for you with goat's cheese! Sometimes I order a big double salad with a bunch of vegetable sides, like sautéed spinach, mushrooms or asparagus, along with a vegetarian soup. I can always find something! No matter what you do, don't order fruit for dessert or a dessert that contains fruit. And don't forget to take your digestive enzymes right before!

4 | **Cleanse on an Ongoing Basis.**

It is essential to incorporate probiotics, digestive enzymes, magnesium-oxygen supplements and lots of Probiotic & Enzyme Salad. These are critical to cleansing the body on an ongoing basis so that you can get more beauty nutrients from the healthy foods you're eating. Getting colonics (or doing at-home enemas) is also recommended when possible. What we cleanse out of our body (the sludge) is just as important as what we put into our body. The more raw plant food we eat, the more toxicity gets kicked up, and the more important and beneficial colonics are.

BEAUTY DETOX PORTION GUIDELINES

Below are some general guidelines for portion sizes, but since everyone's genetic makeup, constitution, metabolism, exercise routine and weight are different, it is key to individualize your diet and portion sizes.

FOOD	AMOUNT
Raw Greens, Non-Starchy Vegetables	Unlimited quantities
Cooked Non-Starchy Vegetables (steamed, baked or lightly sautéed with little or no oil)	Unlimited quantities
Fruit	As we become more alkaline, 3 to 4 servings a day is ideal. Green drinks count as 2 to 3 servings, depending on how much is drank over the course of the day.
Starchy Vegetables	Consume 1 to 1½ cups per day if you are trying to lose weight or maintain your weight and have had difficulty in the past. Many people can have more than one serving by cutting out refined starches and sticking to these starchy vegetables. Individualize your portion size to your activity level and metabolic needs.
Alkaline Grains	Limit to 1 to 1½ cups (cooked) per day if you are trying to lose weight or maintain your weight and have had difficulty in the past. Some people can have more than one serving by cutting out refined grains and starches and sticking to these whole grains. Individualize your portion size to your activity level and metabolic needs.
Ground Flaxseed	Have 1 (or 2, depending on your size) tablespoon daily, sprinkled on salad.

FOOD	AMOUNT
Nuts	Limit to 1 ounce if you are trying to lose weight. Limit to 2 to 3 ounces daily maximum as a general recommendation. Serving size can increase for active people, athletes, children or those trying to gain weight.
Oil	Avoid altogether if you are trying to lose weight. Restrict to 1 tablespoon a day maximum. When cooking, use limited amounts of coconut oil or grapeseed oil, or lower the temperature and simply use a bit of water or vegetable broth instead.
Meat, Fish and Goat's Cheese	Limit to 2 to 3 ounces maximum a serving. Consume at most once a day, at dinner, and work toward a maximum total of 2 to 3 servings a week.

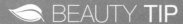 BEAUTY **TIP**

Pick Your Poison

While all alcohol should be limited, I know that it is *not* realistic that all of us will never have a drop of alcohol for the rest of our lives! So the trick is to choose wisely.

Wine is okay in moderation, since it has flavonoids and antioxidants. Choose organic or biodynamic wines with no added sulfites. Though it is fermented and does contain sugar, wine is not as hard on the liver as hard alcohol.

The worst and most toxic drinks are the brewed alcoholic ones, like beer, tequila and rum, which cause sugar imbalances in the body and bloating. If you really want a cocktail, stick to vodka. And if you happen to *really* love your occasional beer (like on Saint Paddy's Day!), at least choose a darker variety, which has more minerals, over refined, lighter-colored varieties. The carbohydrates in dark beers are absorbed more slowly into the bloodstream, so they have a less upsetting effect on your blood sugar level.

YOUR BEAUTY DETOX KITCHEN

You won't need too many new kitchen appliances to get started, but there are a few essentials. Even though you might have to invest in a few new kitchen tools, the investment will come back to you a hundredfold. When we have good equipment, it makes food preparation easier and helps make our food taste better, so we are more inspired to stick with the program. (For additional product options or recommendations other than those listed, you can visit my website at www.kimberlysnyder.net.)

BEAUTY DETOX KITCHEN ESSENTIALS

BLENDER

A good blender is at the top of the list. We'll be using a blender to create the Glowing Green Smoothie and other smoothies, raw soups, salad dressings, nut pâtés and more. A good blender will save you lots of time as it pulverizes food very quickly, efficiently breaking down plant food so its nutrition is readily available for the body without it having to work.

My absolute favorite is the Vitamix. While it is an investment, it will last you forever and is truly invaluable. It is also really easy to clean. You can purchase refurbished ones that were floor models, which are virtually as good as new and come at a much lower cost.

JUICER

We'll be using this to make our Glowing Green Juice. Remember that straight fruit juices are *not* recommended. There are several good juicers I recommend:

Two-Speed Breville Juicer: This is a good basic centrifugal juicer that is easy to clean. Because it is produced from centrifugal motion, juice made from this kind of juicer should ideally be consumed immediately. If you do store juice, be sure to keep it cool and covered, and drink it as soon as you can. The other alternative is freezing individual servings.

Hurom Slow Juicer: This juicer extracts juice by first crushing the plant matter, then squeezing the pulp to extract more juice. This brand of juicer is said to make much more juice than other juicers.

Norwalk Juicer: This is the most superior of all juicers, as it uses a hydraulic press to squeeze juice out of the plant fiber rather than masticating the cell walls, as other juicers do. The main advantage is that the juice oxidizes at a much slower rate, so enzymes are intact for much longer and the juice can be stored longer. The cost is upwards of $2,500.

FOOD PROCESSOR

This is an important kitchen tool that serves different functions than a blender. Food processors are better for mixing ingredients (rather than fully blending or emulsifying them) and are ideal for preparing certain nut pâtés, crusts or anything that needs to retain some texture. If you are on a budget, invest your money into a blender, and you can think of adding a food processor down the line. My favorite is the Cuisinart.

CUTTING BOARD AND SHARP KNIVES

It is best to keep a separate cutting board reserved only for vegetables and fruit. Sharp knives are an absolute essential and will make your life so much better. I'm not kidding! Be sure to keep your knives sharp with a sharpening stone.

CLEAVER

This large, rectangular-shaped knife is a must for chopping open young coconuts.

SALAD SPINNER

Essential! Soggy salads are just *not* appetizing, and this tool whips all that excess water right off lettuce and other greens. I also use the inner strainer piece to wash my vegetables and fruit when I make the Glowing Green Smoothie or the Glowing Green Juice.

MEASURING CUPS AND SPOONS

The Beauty Detox recipes are all basic, but a set of measuring cups and spoons will help ensure you're getting the ingredients and flavors just right.

FINE MESH STRAINER

This is useful for straining quick nut milks, as well as draining our alkaline grains, like quinoa and millet.

CHEESECLOTH

This is useful for straining nut milk. You yield more nut milk when you use cheesecloth than when you use a strainer.

MANDOLINE

This tool is not necessary, but it's nice for slicing vegetables very thin and to a uniform width.

DEHYDRATOR

There are no dehydrated food recipes in this book, as we are now focusing on eating simple fresh food full of water, along with some healthy whole grains. A dehydrator is simply a box with a fan and a small electric heater, in which food is laid on trays. It slowly "bakes" the moisture out of food over many hours, creating raw breads, crackers, desserts, etc. A dehydrator is useful if you want to make creative raw food recipes that require more time, but is certainly not necessary. If you are interested, the Excalibur brand is a good one.

YOUR BEAUTY DETOX SHOPPING LIST

The products listed below are available at your local grocery stores, health markets and farmers' markets. Be sure to buy local and organic products whenever possible!

Fruit and vegetables should be purchased seasonally, and according to your taste. Below is only a *basic* fruit and vegetable list, and it includes certain staples for salads and green drinks.

Before you start shopping, go through your kitchen pantry and cabinets and discard anything that is not Beauty Detox friendly. It might seem like a lot—table salt; balsamic vinegar; dusty old spices; canned, salty vegetables—and that's okay. Remember that these foods are not serving a purpose for you anymore. We are on to better and powerful beauty foods! Check labels if you are not sure, and throw out anything that has foreign chemicals, additives and preservatives. It is time to clean house to make room for our new and improved lifestyle!

The list below is not an exhaustive list, nor is it a required shopping list. But it will give you an idea of how you can stock your new Beauty Detox kitchen. You may even have some of these items already.

Be sure to keep things organized and clean. Organize your spices, dry foods and produce. Keep nuts and seeds in airtight containers, and refrigerate them if you have enough room. The cleaner and more organized your kitchen is, the more enjoyable it will be for you to prepare and enjoy food!

CONDIMENTS, OILS AND SWEETENERS

- ○ Raw, unrefined apple cider vinegar
- ○ Unrefined, raw coconut oil
- ○ Grapeseed oil
- ○ First cold-pressed extra-virgin olive oil
- ○ Celtic or Himalayan sea salt
- ○ Stone-ground or Dijon mustard
- ○ Low sodium tamari
- ○ Nama shoyu unpasteurized soy sauce (contains gluten)
- ○ Organic, unpasteurized (if possible) miso paste
- ○ Bragg Liquid Aminos
- ○ Nutritional yeast
- ○ Raw cacao
- ○ Raw tahini
- ○ Stevia (powdered and liquid) or Xylitol
- ○ Raw honey (optional and for occasional use; not vegan; contains fructose)
- ○ Dried figs and dates (optional and for occasional use)
- ○ Vanilla extract
- ○ Unsweetened almond or hemp milk (unless you always make your own)

ALKALINE GRAINS

- ○ Amaranth
- ○ Buckwheat (kasha)
- ○ Millet
- ○ Quinoa
- ○ Gluten-free products made of grains above, including breads, crackers, cereals, etc.

SEA VEGETABLES

- ○ Arame
- ○ Dulse flakes or chunks
- ○ Kelp
- ○ Nori wrappers
- ○ Wakame

BASIC SPICES

- ○ Black pepper
- ○ Cajun spice (I love this spice blend! Be sure to get a non-salt-containing variety.)
- ○ Cayenne pepper
- ○ Cinnamon
- ○ Coriander
- ○ Cumin
- ○ Curry powder
- ○ Dill, dried
- ○ Italian seasoning
- ○ Oregano
- ○ Paprika

○ Rosemary, dried

○ Turmeric

RAW AND UNSALTED NUTS AND SEEDS

○ Almonds

○ Flaxseeds

○ Hemp seeds

○ Macadamia nuts

○ Pecans

○ Pine nuts

○ Pumpkin seeds

○ Sunflower seeds

○ Walnuts

○ Young coconuts

ALGAE

○ Chlorella (tablets)

○ Spirulina

BASIC FRUITS, VEGETABLES AND HERBS

Remember to choose your fruits and vegetables based on what is local and seasonal.

○ Acai berries (sold frozen at the supermarket)

○ Apples

○ Arugula

○ Avocados

○ Bananas

○ Basil

○ Blueberries

○ Cabbage (weekly essential for Probiotic & Enzyme Salad)

○ Celery

○ Cilantro

○ Collard greens

○ Cucumber

○ Dill

○ Kale

○ Lemons

○ Limes

○ Mustard greens

○ Nectarines

○ Onions

○ Oranges

○ Papaya

○ Parsley

○ Pears

○ Plums

○ Raspberries

○ Red leaf lettuce

○ Romaine lettuce

○ Spinach

○ Sprouts (sunflower, clover, etc.)

○ Strawberries

○ Swiss chard

○ Tomatoes

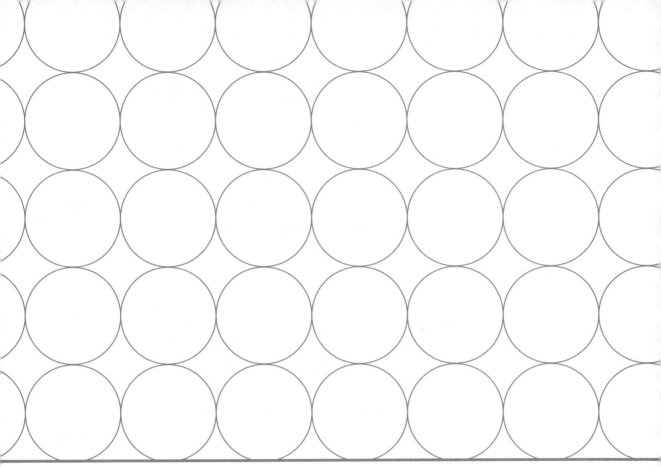

CHAPTER EIGHT

PHASE 1: BLOSSOMING BEAUTY

Health, contentment and trust
Are your greatest possessions,
And freedom your greatest joy.

—Buddha

This plan proves that it *is* possible for *anyone* to make improvements in his or her health—starting right now! You won't have to buy any new kitchen equipment, and many of the foods are upgraded variations of foods with which you are already familiar. In the Blossoming Beauty phase, you can make improvements without starting *too* fast. Before long, you'll experience a newfound confidence and natural glow!

I've introduced many working mothers, busy executives and people that had never been able to stick to a "diet" in the past to the Blossoming Beauty phase, and I have seen amazing results! This plan is appropriate for those that are fifty or more pounds overweight, have candida, are exhausted and don't know where to start.

BLOSSOMING BEAUTY BENEFITS

During this phase, you will be pleased to notice that you are dropping excess pounds and balancing back to your naturally perfect weight, but it is in a steady way that will last for the long term. Unlike when you've lost weight on other programs, you will actually find your energy *increasing* and staying steady through the day. Digestive problems, as well as chronic gassiness and bloat, will abate or disappear completely! As you consume much larger salads and amounts of plant foods, I think you will surprise yourself that you don't need the animal products like you once might have thought you did to stay satiated.

For my friends that have or suspect they have candida, you will be relieved to see that the extreme trouble you may have experienced for many years, such as excess pounds, bloat, gassiness, chronic yeast infections, feeling exhausted all the time and moodiness, will be greatly relieved! Remember that this is a process, as it takes time for the body to rebalance and heal, but you will start to see that recovery is in sight, and within your grasp.

When to Cut Gluten Out Completely

For those that have or suspect they have candida, gluten must be cut out completely. Switch to the other grains and grain products discussed in the Beauty Grains and Starches section on page 111. It is not as hard as you think, and you will be so happy with how much better you feel!

BLOSSOMING BEAUTY BASIC TENETS

○ Since we are working to rebalance our sugar, get rid of carbohydrate cravings, and correct any yeast imbalances, as a Blossoming Beauty, you should avoid:

Fruit (except non-sweet fruit, such as lemons, limes, tomatoes, avocados and cucumbers), including all fruit juice

Dairy

Gluten-containing foods, such as wheat, rye and barley (reduce these to a maximum of three to four times a week rather than completely avoiding them if you must)

Refined sugar and starches, including sodas

Artificial sweeteners, including all diet sodas

Canned and microwaved foods

Unfermented soy products

Foods with additives or artificial ingredients, including packaged foods and pre-bottled fruit and vegetable juices

Table salt

Fried foods

Alcohol (the sugars in it can feed yeast; later a moderate amount of alcohol can be enjoyed occasionally)

Refined or heated oils (except a small amount of coconut oil)

Other oils (even olive oil, unless you are underweight)

○ No animal protein during the day, which slows the passage of food. We stay light and eat only plant-based foods.

○ Minimize snacking as much as possible. Snacking drains our Beauty Energy and overtaxes our system. Eat enough at meals so you feel satisfied and not hungry.

○ If hunger persists through the afternoon because you are used to eating heavier foods or more often, try eating more Probiotic & Enzyme Salad. You should always have veggies sticks around to snack on with salsa or another veggie-based dip. Chlorella tablets can also be helpful.

○ Nuts can be consumed in a quantity of one ounce or less per day. Eating more than one ounce during this phase will be too heavy and concentrated and may hinder your progress.

○ Dinner is vegetarian at least three times a week.

Since you are just starting out, there *may* be times when, because of your cravings, your emotions, what is going on in your life or some other reason, you miscombine and resort to your old favorite foods. To counterbalance this, increase the size of your big predinner green salad with oil-free dressing. Remember the seesaw? The heavier the food you are going to eat next (lasagna with meat), the bigger your oil-free salad better be! The salad, full of water and fiber, will help absorb some of the really bad, dense foods. The salad helps keep the seesaw in balance as much as possible, even when we are "cheating."

BLOSSOMING BEAUTY SAMPLE ONE-WEEK MENU

○ Meals for any day can be interchanged with a *lighter* meal (for example, Dharma's Kale Salad instead of an Open-Faced Avo Beauty Sandwich), but not the other way around.

○ This plan is meant to be a guide, so be sure to customize your meals accordingly. Of course, I don't expect you to make all these recipes every week. There will be really easy dishes you love and can make effortlessly and without thinking. That is wonderful! Keep it simple. You can also enjoy leftovers when you have them.

How Long Should You Be a Blossoming Beauty?

If you have a serious candida or sugar issue, you may need to stick with the Blossoming Beauty phase for three months. After this time period, you can see if you have cleansed your body enough or starved the yeast enough to handle fruit.

To do so, take the "fruit challenge" that Dr. William G. Crook describes in *The Yeast Connection and Women's Health.*[1] He says to take a small bite of fruit and wait ten minutes to see if there is a negative reaction. If not, take another bite. If there are no adverse reactions for an hour, finish the piece of fruit. The best fruits to start reintroducing into the system are the sour fruits grapefruit and kiwi. Dr. Edward Howell, in his book *Enzyme Nutrition,*

recommends a similar approach—starting with a small amount of fruit and slowing increasing the quantity until moderate amounts of fruit can be tolerated comfortably.[2]

In the Radiant Beauty phase, we start to reintroduce fruit. When you transition, carefully monitor how you feel as you start to reintroduce fruit. If you still experience adverse symptoms to fruit (bloating or any form of digestive discomfort), drop back to Blossoming Beauty and try again in a few weeks or when you feel ready. As our bodies become more alkaline and clean, we will thrive off fruit and digest fruit wonderfully, and fruit will become one of our most important allies in our quest for true beauty!

○ Be sure to refer to the Beauty Detox Portion Guidelines (page 159) to be familiar with how much of certain foods to eat.

○ If you get a craving for dessert, especially while transitioning, herbal tea or warmed unsweetened almond milk with stevia might satisfy you. One to two ounces of an organic, 72 percent or more cacao, dairy-free dark chocolate bar is another choice, though we do not want to consume chocolate every day. If you're really craving something sweet, you can try some of the smoothie and dessert recipes (ones that don't have nuts or dried fruits) in Chapter 11. Some good options are the Rain Forest Acai Smoothie, Happy Cow Dairy-Free Hot Chocolate and Chia Seed Delight.

○ Add one tablespoon of ground flaxseed to your dinner salad every day to satisfy your omega-3 essential fatty acid needs.

○ Having a cup of hot water with liver-supporting lemon first thing in the morning supports our cleansing process.

FIRST THING	A cup of hot water with the juice of half a lemon One probiotic supplement with one full pint of water	DAY ONE
BREAKFAST (always the same)	Two or three celery stalks Followed by Raw Rolled Oat Cereal or one to two pieces of toasted, plain gluten-free sprouted millet bread (with a small amount of organic butter, if necessary)	
LUNCH	Start with a digestive enzyme Large serving of Dharma's Kale Salad Followed by a large bowl of minestrone soup or Delish Squash Bisque, along with a handful of gluten-free crackers (optional)	
SNACK (at least thee hours later)	Veggie sticks dipped in Sally's Salsa	
DINNER	Start with a digestive enzyme Large green salad with Oil-Free Red Pepper and Cilantro Dressing and ½ cup of Probiotic & Enzyme Salad Followed by lightly steamed broccoli and a piece of baked fish with lemon, or an Alkaline-Grain Veggie Burger	
LATE NIGHT	If you experience cravings, have herbal tea with stevia or more veggie sticks dipped in Sally's Salsa or Green Bean–Miso Dip	
BEFORE BED	One probiotic supplement Two to four capsules of a magnesium-oxygen supplement, as needed	

DAY TWO		
FIRST THING	A cup of hot water with the juice of half a lemon One probiotic supplement with one full pint of water	
BREAKFAST (always the same)	Two or three celery stalks Followed by Raw Rolled Oat Cereal or one to two pieces of toasted, plain gluten-free sprouted millet bread (with a small amount of organic butter, if necessary)	
LUNCH	Start with a digestive enzyme Large romaine salad with Oil-Free/Balsamic-Free Italian Vinaigrette Dressing Followed by the Open-Faced Avo Beauty Sandwich	
SNACK (at least thee hours later)	Veggie sticks dipped in Raw Chickpea-Less Hummus	
DINNER	Start with a digestive enzyme Large mixed green salad with Kim's Classic Dressing and ½ cup of Probiotic & Enzyme Salad Followed by one to two cups of lightly sautéed spinach with garlic and coconut oil, and baked or roasted chicken, or Greek-Inspired Millet Salad	
LATE NIGHT	If you experience cravings, have herbal tea with stevia or more veggie sticks dipped in Sally's Salsa or Green Bean–Miso Dip	
BEFORE BED	One probiotic supplement Two to four capsules of a magnesium-oxygen supplement, as needed	

DAY THREE		
FIRST THING	A cup of hot water with the juice of half a lemon One probiotic supplement with one full pint of water	
BREAKFAST (always the same)	Two or three celery stalks Followed by Raw Rolled Oat Cereal or one to two pieces of toasted, plain gluten-free sprouted millet bread (with a small amount of organic butter, if necessary)	
LUNCH	Large mixed green salad with Asian Miso-Carrot Dressing and ½ cup of Probiotic & Enzyme Salad Followed by Fresh Romaine Soft Tacos	
SNACK (at least thee hours later)	Veggie sticks dipped in ½ cup of Beauty Guacamole	
DINNER	Start with a digestive enzyme Dharma's Kale Salad and ½ cup of Probiotic & Enzyme Salad Followed by Veggie-Turmeric Quinoa	
LATE NIGHT	If you experience cravings, have herbal tea with stevia or more veggie sticks dipped in Sally's Salsa or Green Bean–Miso Dip	
BEFORE BED	One probiotic supplement Two to four capsules of a magnesium-oxygen supplement, as needed	

FIRST THING	A cup of hot water with the juice of half a lemon One probiotic supplement with one full pint of water
BREAKFAST (always the same)	Two or three celery stalks Followed by Raw Rolled Oat Cereal or one to two pieces of toasted, plain gluten-free sprouted millet bread (with a small amount of organic butter, if necessary)
LUNCH	Large serving of Spirulina Spinach Salad or Dharma's Kale Salad
SNACK (at least thee hours later)	Celery sticks with ½ cup Raw Chickpea-Less Hummus
DINNER	Start with a digestive enzyme Large serving of Sunday Salad and ½ cup of Probiotic & Enzyme Salad Followed by quinoa pasta topped with an organic marinara sauce and vegetables or Rainbow Stuffed Peppers
LATE NIGHT	If you experience cravings, have herbal tea with stevia or more veggie sticks dipped in Sally's Salsa or Green Bean–Miso Dip
BEFORE BED	One probiotic supplement Two to four capsules of a magnesium-oxygen supplement, as needed

FIRST THING	A cup of hot water with the juice of half a lemon One probiotic supplement with one full pint of water
BREAKFAST (always the same)	Two or three celery stalks Followed by Raw Rolled Oat Cereal or one to two pieces of toasted, plain gluten-free sprouted millet bread (with a small amount of organic butter, if necessary)
LUNCH	Start with a digestive enzyme Large mixed green salad with Oil-Free Red Pepper and Cilantro Dressing Followed by the Open-Faced Avo Beauty Sandwich
SNACK (at least thee hours later)	Veggie sticks with Green Bean–Miso Dip
DINNER	Start with a digestive enzyme Large serving of Dharma's Kale Salad and ½ cup of Probiotic & Enzyme Salad Followed by one to two cups lightly steamed vegetables topped with lemon and a dash of Celtic sea salt, and some poached wild Alaskan salmon, or a veggie omelet with two organic eggs or Millet "Couscous" Salad
LATE NIGHT	If you experience cravings, have herbal tea with stevia or more veggie sticks dipped in Sally's Salsa or Green Bean–Miso Dip
BEFORE BED	One probiotic supplement Two to four capsules of a magnesium-oxygen supplement, as needed

DAY SIX		
FIRST THING	A cup of hot water with the juice of half a lemon One probiotic supplement with one full pint of water
BREAKFAST (always the same)	Two or three celery stalks Followed by Raw Rolled Oat Cereal or one to two pieces of toasted, plain gluten-free sprouted millet bread (with a small amount of organic butter, if necessary)
LUNCH	Start with a digestive enzyme Large green salad with Dreamy Creamy Avocado Dressing Followed by one to two cups of East-West Baked Vegetables
SNACK (at least thee hours later)	Veggie sticks with Green Bean–Miso Dip
DINNER	Start with a digestive enzyme Large green salad with Oil-Free/Balsamic-Free Italian Vinaigrette Dressing and ½ cup of Probiotic & Enzyme Salad Followed by lightly steamed broccoli and a piece of baked fish with lemon, or Raw Tabouli Salad with Hemp Seeds topped with two hardboiled organic eggs
LATE NIGHT	If you experience cravings, have herbal tea with stevia or more veggie sticks dipped in Sally's Salsa or Green Bean–Miso Dip
BEFORE BED	One probiotic supplement Two to four capsules of a magnesium-oxygen supplement, as needed

DAY SEVEN		
FIRST THING	A cup of hot water with the juice of half a lemon One probiotic supplement with one full pint of water
BREAKFAST (always the same)	Two or three celery stalks Followed by Raw Rolled Oat Cereal or one to two pieces of toasted, plain gluten-free sprouted millet bread (with a small amount of organic butter, if necessary)
LUNCH	Israeli Chopped Salad followed by the Ananda Burrito
SNACK (at least thee hours later)	Veggie sticks dipped in ½ cup of Beauty Guacamole
DINNER	Start with a digestive enzyme Large serving of Sunday Salad and ½ cup of Probiotic & Enzyme Salad Followed by Quinoa, Avocado and Corn Salad
LATE NIGHT	If you experience cravings, have herbal tea with stevia or more veggie sticks dipped in Sally's Salsa or Green Bean–Miso Dip
BEFORE BED	One probiotic supplement Two to four capsules of a magnesium-oxygen supplement, as needed

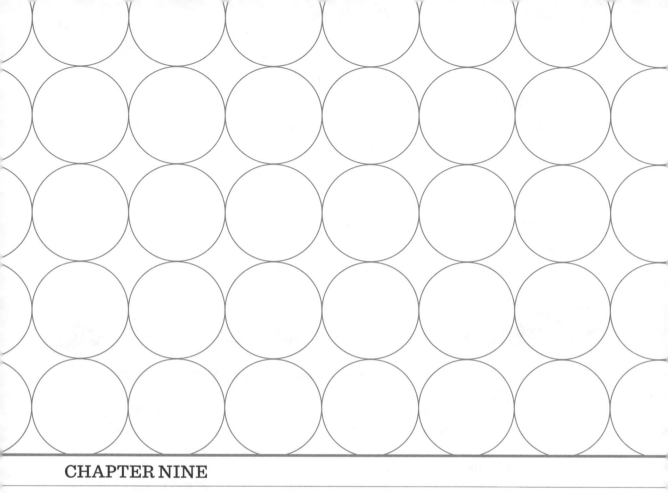

CHAPTER NINE

PHASE 2: RADIANT BEAUTY

Determine now to break out of the jail of habits and race for freedom.

—Paramahansa Yogananda

Becoming a Radiant Beauty is super exciting! We are moving to a higher level of health and beauty and becoming more immersed in the wonderful abundance of fresh, nutrient-dense and beautifying plant foods! In the Radiant Beauty phase we add the Glowing Green Smoothie, which is a powerful weapon that will improve our skin and hair and help us rebalance our weight. Embrace how great the plan makes you look and feel the more you stick with it.

Radiant Beauty adheres to the same tenets as Blossoming Beauty, except we take fruit off the "avoid" list. Oil may be reintroduced in small amounts and your daily serving of nuts can increase from one to two ounces. If you are coming to Radiant Beauty from

What Happens if I Hit a Wall?

It happens to all of us. We are flying high, losing weight easily and rapidly, our skin is looking great, our energy is unbeatable, and then suddenly, boom, everything comes to a screeching halt. Weight loss plateaus. Cravings may start kicking back in. A few zits rear their ugly heads. Along with the physical issues, we may start to mentally beat ourselves up or get really frustrated and ask ourselves, "What am I doing wrong?"

The answer is that probably you are doing nothing wrong. Remember the analogy to the clogged wheel? True and deep cleansing not only takes years, but it is an ongoing process. You will have ups and downs. There may be periods when you bring more waste up to the surface and it is more difficult to get rid of. Maybe you brought a great deal to the surface and now some cravings have set in. You may have slipped up a few times and had a tuna melt or a chicken sandwich. Big deal! Forget about it and move on with the plan! Forward momentum is what we are most concerned with. You don't have to be perfect; you just have to keep focusing on making progress. You know how long it took me to totally forget about cheese and never ever truly want it again? *Two years*. Yes, for two years I struggled to cut it out of my life!

When you get into a rut, it is a good idea to make sure you are taking your magnesium-oxygen supplements, drinking a lot of water and eating very simply. It certainly wouldn't be a bad idea to get a properly administered gravity colonic to move more waste out in an efficient and timely way. Eat really lightly for a day or two, cutting back on even alkaline grain dishes or nut pâtés, and see if that helps you get through.

Most importantly, remember that we all go through periods of flux! This might happen especially around the changes of season, by the way. I go through it too. Be patient with yourself, and remember that this is a lifestyle program, not a temporary diet. Stay positive, don't indulge yourself or be hard on yourself or wallow in your cravings too much, and you will soon get back on track!

Blossoming Beauty, be sure to read the note on transitioning, How Long Should You Be a Blossoming Beauty? on page 170 first.

Get ready to launch into a whole new level of beauty!

RADIANT BEAUTY BENEFITS

Ladies and gentlemen, this is your captain speaking. I'd like to thank you for joining me as we skyrocket toward new levels of health and beauty. En route, we will be crossing over into new frontiers of energy, radiant skin, and lustrous hair and shedding excess pounds in possibly the greatest phase of weight loss. Once we have reached our cruising altitude and stabilized over the next thirty days or so, we will turn off the seat-belt indicator and let you move freely through your life…much more healthy and beautiful, and free of calorie counting and carb counting! I'd like to thank you for joining me, and I hope that in the future, when you need a beauty and health boost, you'll remember to come back to the tenets of the Radiant Beauty phase and remember your secret weapon: the Glowing Green Smoothie!

Since we have increased our fresh greens intake even more with the Glowing Green Smoothie and cut out acid-forming foods further, you may notice, if you are overweight or looking to lose a significant amount of weight, that this is the phase where you experience the highest levels of weight loss. Though you may be skeptical that one little smoothie—the Glowing Green Smoothie—could do so much, you will surprise yourself at how much energy you have from drinking it, and you will feel so good that you won't miss your old breakfast foods over time. You might start going to the bathroom quite a bit more than you were previously used to, which is a great sign that you are starting to dislodge some of the old sludge.

You may notice much bigger differences in your skin, in that it is clearer, softer and more vibrant. It usually takes a few months to see a difference in your hair and your nails, but shinier, thicker hair is on the way and stronger nails to boot!

RADIANT BEAUTY BASIC TENETS

In this phase you will enjoy the Glowing Green Smoothie in the mornings and will start to keep your mornings even lighter to promote cleansing. Many of the other principles are exactly the same as for Blossoming Beauty, except that we work to further reduce the acid-forming animal products in our diet and to cut gluten out completely.

IN THE RADIANT BEAUTY PHASE:

○ The Glowing Green Smoothie will be breakfast at least five times a week. The other days breakfast will be fresh fruit.

○ Cooked foods or grains are not consumed in the morning.

○ Animal products, including land animals, dairy, fish, eggs and raw goat's cheese, are limited to a maximum of three times a week, at dinner only.

○ Dinner is vegetarian at least four times a week.

APPLICABLE TO ALL PHASES:

○ Avoid these foods:

Dairy

Gluten-containing foods, such as those made with wheat, rye and barley

Refined sugar and starches, including all sodas

Artificial sweeteners, including all diet sodas

Canned and microwaved foods

Unfermented soy products

Foods with additives or artificial ingredients; packaged foods

Packaged, pre-bottled fruit and vegetable juices

Table salt

Fried foods

Refined or heated oils (except a small amount of coconut oil)

○ Avoid animal protein during the day, which slows the passage of food. Stay light and eat only plant-based foods.

○ Minimize snacking as much as possible. Snacking drains our Beauty Energy and overtaxes our system. Eat enough at meals so you feel satisfied and not hungry.

○ If hunger persists through the afternoon because you are used to eating heavier foods or eating more often, try having more Probiotic & Enzyme Salad. Have veggie sticks around to snack on with salsa or another veggie-based dip. Chlorella tablets can also be helpful.

How Long Should You Be a Radiant Beauty?

This is arguably the biggest transition of any phase, as we are introducing the Glowing Green Smoothie. This starts to really rebalance the body in a stronger way, due to its fiber and high chlorophyll levels. So don't rush yourself in the adjustment process! The bare minimum is thirty days. But the reality is that making it to the Radiant Beauty phase is a big deal! You should be extremely proud of yourself for making such changes to improve your beauty and health simultaneously. You are having a Glowing Green Smoothie nearly every day, which has totally changed your diet for the whole first part of your day! You have now given up dairy and gluten products (at least most of the time!). Your intake of animal products has been cut way down.

Though you may not be a total vegetarian, you have acid-forming animal products only several times a week. While I personally choose to refrain from all animal products (except occasionally honey), I understand that for familial, cultural or social reasons that may not be 100 percent realistic or possible for all of us.

Since these are huge changes, most of my clients stay in this phase for many months, while some stay in it for years, and some stay in it forever. If it works for you, I fully encourage you to stay with it! Not everyone will move up to the True Beauty phase, simply because the Radiant Beauty phase works for them and their lifestyle. And that is okay, because they have already made huge progress!

Of course, this is not to discourage those of you that want to go further with the lifestyle and try the True Beauty phase. But if it doesn't work for you and you want to stay a Radiant Beauty, that is wonderful! Just be sure that the lifestyle feels comfortable and automatic for you, and that you aren't feeling deprived all the time. It is your personal experience of the outstanding results—great physical improvement, feeling better, having more energy—that will truly and naturally push you forward, or inspire you to stick with what you're doing now. Be in tune with yourself, and don't be judgmental or competitive by trying to get "higher" up. Enjoy the great results, no matter where you are and what is working for you!

RADIANT BEAUTY SAMPLE ONE-WEEK MENU

○ Meals for any day can be interchanged with a *lighter* meal (for example, Dharma's Kale Salad instead of an Open-Faced Avo Beauty Sandwich), but not the other way around.

○ This plan is meant to be a guide, so be sure to customize your meals accordingly. Of course, I don't expect you to make all these recipes every week! There will be leftovers, and you'll make really easy dishes on the fly. You'll develop a list of go-to, easy recipes that you'll make often.

○ Be sure to refer to the Beauty Detox Portion Guidelines (page 159) to be familiar with how much of certain foods to eat.

○ If you get a craving for dessert, herbal tea or warmed unsweetened almond milk with stevia might satisfy you. One to two ounces of an organic, 72 percent or more cacao, dairy-free dark chocolate bar is another choice, though you do not want to consume chocolate every day. If you're really craving something sweet, you can try some of the smoothie and dessert recipes in Chapter 11.

○ Be sure to consume one tablespoon of ground flaxseed a day to satisfy your omega-3 essential fatty acid needs. Add it to your dinner salad each night.

○ Having a cup of hot water with liver-supporting lemon first thing in the morning supports our cleansing process.

DAY ONE		
FIRST THING	A cup of hot water with the juice of half a lemon One probiotic supplement with one full pint of water
BREAKFAST (when we really feel hungry)	Sixteen to thirty ounces of the Glowing Green Smoothie Wait twenty minutes, and only if you are still hungry, follow with a small avocado or half of a large avocado
LUNCH	Start with a digestive enzyme Large serving of Dharma's Kale Salad Followed by Raw Red Pepper and Tomato Soup and a handful of gluten-free crackers (optional)
SNACK (optional at least three hours later)	Eight to twenty ounces of the Glowing Green Smoothie or Rain Forest Acai Smoothie
DINNER	Start with a digestive enzyme Large green salad with Oil-Free/Balsamic-Free Italian Vinaigrette Dressing and ½ cup of Probiotic & Enzyme Salad Followed by Beauty Nut Pâté or Macadamia Nut and Sundried Tomato Mash on collard green wraps
BEFORE BED	One probiotic supplement Two to four capsules of a magnesium-oxygen supplement, as needed

FIRST THING	A cup of hot water with the juice of half a lemon One probiotic supplement with one full pint of water	**DAY TWO**
BREAKFAST (when we really feel hungry)	Sixteen to thirty ounces of the Glowing Green Smoothie Wait twenty minutes, and only if you are still hungry, follow with a small avocado or half of a large avocado	
LUNCH	Large green salad with Kim's Classic Dressing Followed by Fresh Romaine Soft Tacos	
SNACK (optional at least three hours later)	Fresh seasonal and organic fruit	
DINNER	Start with a digestive enzyme Large green salad with Oil-Free Red Pepper and Cilantro Dressing and ½ cup of Probiotic & Enzyme Salad Followed by East-West Baked Vegetables and baked fish with lemon or the JMP Raw Lasagna	
BEFORE BED	One probiotic supplement Two to four capsules of a magnesium-oxygen supplement, as needed	

FIRST THING	A cup of hot water with the juice of half a lemon One probiotic supplement with one full pint of water	**DAY THREE**
BREAKFAST (when we really feel hungry)	One full grapefruit (or seasonal fruit) Wait twenty minutes, and only if you are still hungry, follow with a small avocado or half of a large avocado	
LUNCH	Large green salad with Dreamy Creamy Avocado Dressing Followed by the Ananda Burrito or an Open-Faced Avo Beauty Sandwich	
SNACK (optional at least three hours later)	Eight to twenty ounces of the Glowing Green Smoothie	
DINNER	Start with a digestive enzyme Large green salad with Omega-3 Flax Dressing and ½ cup of Probiotic & Enzyme Salad Followed by Veggie-Turmeric Quinoa or Basic Yams with East-West Baked Vegetables	
BEFORE BED	One probiotic supplement Two to four capsules of a magnesium-oxygen supplement, as needed	

DAY FOUR		
	FIRST THING	A cup of hot water with the juice of half a lemon One probiotic supplement with one full pint of water
	BREAKFAST (when we really feel hungry)	Sixteen to thirty ounces of the Glowing Green Smoothie Wait twenty minutes, and only if you are still hungry, follow with a small avocado or half of a large avocado
	LUNCH	Start with a digestive enzyme Large serving of Sunday Salad Followed by Cauliflower Energy Soup and a handful of gluten-free crackers (optional)
	SNACK (optional at least three hours later)	Fresh seasonal and organic fruit
	DINNER	Start with a digestive enzyme Large green salad with Asian Miso-Carrot Dressing, with ½ cup Probiotic & Enzyme Salad Followed by lightly steamed asparagus and baked fish with lemon or veggie omelet made with two organic eggs or an Alkaline-Grain Veggie Burger
	BEFORE BED	One probiotic supplement Two to four capsules of a magnesium-oxygen supplement, as needed

DAY FIVE		
	FIRST THING	A cup of hot water with the juice of half a lemon One probiotic supplement with one full pint of water
	BREAKFAST (when we really feel hungry)	Sixteen to thirty ounces of the Glowing Green Smoothie Wait twenty minutes, and only if you are still hungry, follow with a small avocado or half of a large avocado
	LUNCH	Large bowl of Spirulina Spinach Salad
	SNACK (optional at least three hours later)	Veggie sticks dipped in Sally's Salsa
	DINNER	Start with a digestive enzyme Large green salad with Oil-Free Red Pepper and Cilantro Dressing, with ½ cup Probiotic & Enzyme Salad Followed by Quinoa, Avocado and Corn Salad or Rainbow Stuffed Peppers
	BEFORE BED	One probiotic supplement Two to four capsules of a magnesium-oxygen supplement, as needed

FIRST THING	A cup of hot water with the juice of half a lemon One probiotic supplement with one full pint of water
BREAKFAST (when we really feel hungry)	One whole grapefruit (or seasonal fruit) Wait twenty minutes, and only if you are still hungry, follow with a small avocado or half of a large avocado
LUNCH	Start with a digestive enzyme Large serving of Dharma's Kale Salad Followed by Italian-Style Sweet Potatoes or Ganesha's Sweet Potatoes
SNACK (optional at least three hours later)	Eight to twenty ounces of the Glowing Green Smoothie
DINNER	Start with a digestive enzyme Large green salad with Kim's Classic Dressing, with ½ cup Probiotic & Enzyme Salad Followed by Bruce's Pine Nut Parmesan or Beauty Nut Pâté and sprouts on collard green wraps
BEFORE BED	One probiotic supplement Two to four capsules of a magnesium-oxygen supplement, as needed

FIRST THING	A cup of hot water with the juice of half a lemon One probiotic supplement with one full pint of water
BREAKFAST (when we really feel hungry)	Sixteen to thirty ounces of the Glowing Green Smoothie Wait twenty minutes, and only if you are still hungry, follow with a small avocado or half of a large avocado
LUNCH	Raw Tabouli Salad with Hemp Seeds and a bowl of Cauliflower Energy Soup
SNACK (optional at least three hours later)	Fresh seasonal and organic fruit
DINNER	Start with a digestive enzyme Large serving of Sunday Salad and ½ cup of Probiotic & Enzyme Salad Followed by East-West Baked Vegetables topped with three ounces of raw unpasteurized goat's cheese (optional) or a scoop of Macadamia Nut and Sundried Tomato Mash
BEFORE BED	One probiotic supplement Two to four capsules of a magnesium-oxygen supplement, as needed

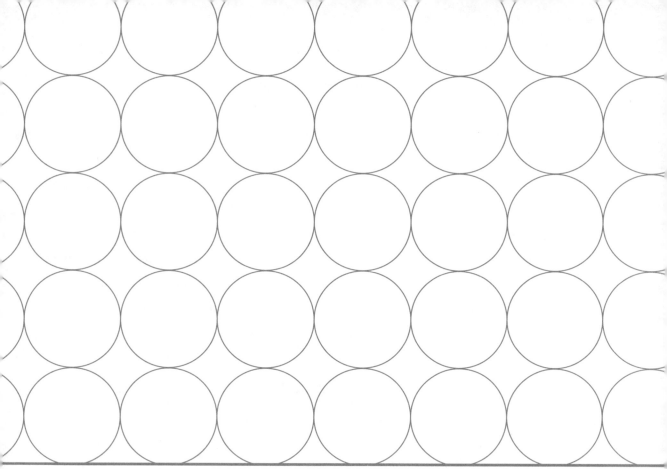

CHAPTER TEN

PHASE 3: TRUE BEAUTY

If you feel bound, you are bound. If you feel liberated, you are liberated. Things outside neither bound nor liberate you; only your attitude toward them does that.

—Sri Swami Satchidananda
Translation and Commentary of the Yoga Sutras of Patanjali

Welcome to True Beauty! True Beauty is a pretty high level of cleansing, and if you have transitioned here, you should be very proud of yourself.

By now you're already starting to see the incredible benefits of the Beauty Detox. Those dark circles under your eyes have lightened. Your skin looks smoother and more radiant. Your eyes are brighter. Your energy level has increased. You may even feel less stressed thanks to the nourishing minerals and nutrients coursing through your body!

As a True Beauty, you'll deepen your cleanse even further, reaching a new level of health and beauty. The longer you stay a True Beauty, the better you will feel and look. Remember the clogged wheel and our theory that aging is essentially only a function of how much sludge we have in our "wheel"? Well, in this phase we reach an exceptionally high level of cleaning out the sludge, reversing aging and growing younger!

TRUE BEAUTY BENEFITS

During this phase, your weight will stabilize and you will achieve the right weight for your frame. You will notice that parts of your body, such as your arms, will become more toned as a result of having more space for the oxygen to move around in your body.

Because you are cleansing and renewing your body at such a high level, you will notice that old nagging cravings will greatly diminish and then will go away, as "reminders" of old foods finally leave your body once and for all, and you restore inner balance in your body. The healthy bacteria in your body are replenished, and your entire body becomes more alkaline. You will not miss old foods or your old lifestyle. You will be so psyched by how great you look and feel! Instead of seeing isolated improvements here and there in your physical features, you will now look in the mirror and increasingly see a more glowing, younger version of yourself. You will experience for yourself the truth of how powerful food and cleansing really are to heal the body and naturally elevate our beauty to its highest level!

Ultimate health and beauty are yours for the taking!

TRUE BEAUTY BASIC TENETS

In True Beauty, we switch from the Glowing Green Smoothie to the Glowing Green Juice. Since we are taking fiber out of the morning routine, we are starting to live on pure plant fuel. The antioxidants and cleansing force in the Glowing Green Juice hit our system in a harder way. If you don't feel comfortable with this, especially at first, don't judge yourself! If at any point in this phase you start to feel like it is too much, return to Radiant Beauty for a while, until you feel like trying again.

If you prefer the Glowing Green Smoothie over the Glowing Green Juice and feel better drinking it (many of my clients do), you can definitely stick with it but adhere to the other tenets of the plan. The Glowing Green Smoothie can also be a snack later on in the day, after lunch, even if you have Glowing Green Juice in the morning.

IN THE TRUE BEAUTY PHASE:

- The Glowing Green Juice will be breakfast at least five times a week (unless you find that you do better on the Glowing Green Smoothie and choose to stick with it).
- Lunch no longer includes any cooked grains. Cooked veggies and avocados are the densest solid foods at lunch.
- Fish and other seafood, eggs and raw goat's milk cheese are consumed a maximum of two times a week at dinner. All other meals have no animal products.
- Land animals (chicken, beef, pork, turkey, etc.) are no longer consumed.

APPLICABLE TO ALL PHASES:

- Avoid these foods:

Dairy	Unfermented soy products
Gluten-containing foods, such as those made with wheat, rye and barley	Packaged, pre-bottled fruit and vegetable juices
Refined sugar and starches, including sodas	Table salt
Artificial sweeteners, including all diet sodas	Fried foods
Canned and microwaved foods	Refined or heated oils (except a small amount of coconut oil)
Foods with additives or artificial ingredients; packaged foods	

- Avoid animal protein during the day, which slows the passage of food. Stay light and eat only plant-based foods.

○ Minimize snacking as much as possible. Snacking drains our Beauty Energy and overtaxes our system. Eat enough at meals so you feel satisfied and not hungry.

○ If hunger persists through the afternoon because you are used to eating heavier foods or more often, try eating more Probiotic & Enzyme Salad. Have veggie sticks around to snack on with salsa or another veggie-based dip. Chlorella tablets can also be helpful.

TRUE BEAUTY SAMPLE ONE-WEEK MENU

○ Meals for any day can be interchanged with a *lighter* meal (for example, Dharma's Kale Salad instead of an Open-Faced Avo Beauty Sandwich), but not the other way around.

○ This plan is meant to be a guide, so be sure to customize your meals accordingly. Of course, I don't expect you to make all these recipes every week! There will be leftovers, and you'll make really easy dishes on the fly. You'll develop a list of go-to, easy recipes that you'll make often!

○ Be sure to refer to the Beauty Detox Portion Guidelines (page 159) to be familiar with how much of certain foods to eat.

○ If you get a craving for dessert, herbal tea or warmed unsweetened almond milk with stevia might satisfy you. One to two ounces of an organic, 72 percent or more cacao, dairy-free dark chocolate bar is another choice, though you do not want to consume chocolate every day. If you're really craving something sweet, you can try some of the smoothie and dessert recipes in Chapter 11.

○ Be sure to consume one tablespoon of ground flaxseed a day to satisfy your need for omega-3 essential fatty acid needs. Add it to your dinner salad each night.

○ Having a cup of hot water with liver-supporting lemon first thing in the morning supports our cleansing process.

FIRST THING	A cup of hot water with the juice of half a lemon One probiotic supplement with one full pint of water
BREAKFAST (when we really feel hungry)	Sixteen to thirty-two ounces of the Glowing Green Juice Wait twenty minutes, and only if you are still hungry, follow with a piece of fruit or the Glowing Green Smoothie
LUNCH	Large bowl of Dharma's Kale Salad
SNACK (optional at least three hours later)	Eight to twenty ounces of the Glowing Green Smoothie
DINNER	Start with a digestive enzyme Large green salad with Omega-3 Flax Dressing and ½ cup of Probiotic & Enzyme Salad Followed by the Alkaline-Grain Veggie Burger
BEFORE BED	One probiotic supplement Two to four capsules of a magnesium-oxygen supplement, as needed

FIRST THING	A cup of hot water with the juice of half a lemon One probiotic supplement with one full pint of water
BREAKFAST (when we really feel hungry)	Sixteen to thirty-two ounces of the Glowing Green Juice Wait twenty minutes, and only if you are still hungry, follow with a piece of fruit or the Glowing Green Smoothie
LUNCH	Large green salad with Kim's Classic Dressing Followed by the Ananda Burrito
SNACK (optional at least three hours later)	Eight to twenty ounces of the Glowing Green Smoothie or veggie sticks with Sally's Salsa
DINNER	Start with a digestive enzyme Large bowl of Dharma's Kale Salad or Sunday Salad Followed by Italian-Style Sweet Potatoes or Ganesha's Sweet Potatoes
BEFORE BED	One probiotic supplement Two to four capsules of a magnesium-oxygen supplement, as needed

DAY THREE		
FIRST THING	A cup of hot water with the juice of half a lemon One probiotic supplement with one full pint of water	
BREAKFAST (when we really feel hungry)	Sixteen to thirty-two ounces of the Glowing Green Juice Wait twenty minutes, and only if you are still hungry, follow with a piece of fruit or the Glowing Green Smoothie	
LUNCH	A large bowl of Spirulina Spinach Salad Followed by the Avo-Tomato Lunch Plate	
SNACK (optional at least three hours later)	Eight to twenty ounces of the Glowing Green Smoothie or the Thirty-Second Spirulina Superfood Drink	
DINNER	Start with a digestive enzyme Green salad with Oil-Free Red Pepper and Cilantro Dressing and ½ cup of Probiotic & Enzyme Salad Followed by lightly steamed broccoli and a piece of baked fish with lemon or the Quinoa, Avocado and Corn Salad or the JMP Raw Lasagna	
BEFORE BED	One probiotic supplement Two to four capsules of a magnesium-oxygen supplement, as needed	

DAY FOUR		
FIRST THING	A cup of hot water with the juice of half a lemon One probiotic supplement with one full pint of water	
BREAKFAST (when we really feel hungry)	Sixteen to thirty-two ounces of the Glowing Green Juice Wait twenty minutes, and only if you are still hungry, follow with a piece of fruit or the Glowing Green Smoothie	
LUNCH	Large serving of green salad with Asian Miso-Carrot Dressing Followed by a bowl of Cauliflower Energy Soup	
SNACK (optional at least three hours later)	Eight to twenty ounces of the Glowing Green Smoothie	
DINNER	Start with a digestive enzyme Large serving of Sunday Salad and ½ cup of Probiotic & Enzyme Salad topped with one scoop of Bruce's Pine Nut Parmesan or three ounces of raw goat's cheese	
BEFORE BED	One probiotic supplement Two to four capsules of a magnesium-oxygen supplement, as needed	

DAY FIVE		
FIRST THING	A cup of hot water with the juice of half a lemon One probiotic supplement with one full pint of water	
BREAKFAST (when we really feel hungry)	Sixteen to thirty-two ounces of the Glowing Green Juice Wait twenty minutes, and only if you are still hungry, follow with a piece of fruit or the Glowing Green Smoothie	
LUNCH	Israeli Chopped Salad Followed by Fresh Romaine Soft Tacos	
SNACK (optional at least three hours later)	Eight to twenty ounces of the Glowing Green Smoothie or a piece of fruit	
DINNER	Start with a digestive enzyme Large serving of green salad with Oil-Free/Balsamic-Free Italian Vinaigrette Dressing Followed by a veggie omelet made with two organic eggs or Veggie-Turmeric Quinoa or a scoop of Macadamia Nut and Sundried Tomato Mash	
BEFORE BED	One probiotic supplement Two to four capsules of a magnesium-oxygen supplement, as needed	

DAY SIX		
FIRST THING	A cup of hot water with the juice of half a lemon One probiotic supplement with one full pint of water	
BREAKFAST (when we really feel hungry)	Sixteen to thirty-two ounces of the Glowing Green Juice Wait twenty minutes, and only if you are still hungry, follow with a piece of fruit or the Glowing Green Smoothie	
LUNCH	Large serving of green salad with Dreamy Creamy Avocado Dressing Followed by a bowl of Raw Red Pepper and Tomato Soup	
SNACK (optional at least three hours later)	Eight to twenty ounces of the Glowing Green Smoothie	
DINNER	Start with a digestive enzyme Large serving of green salad with Oil-Free/Balsamic-Free Italian Vinaigrette Dressing Followed by Greek-Inspired Millet Salad or Rainbow Stuffed Peppers	
BEFORE BED	One probiotic supplement Two to four capsules of a magnesium-oxygen supplement, as needed	

DAY SEVEN		
	FIRST THING	A cup of hot water with the juice of half a lemon One probiotic supplement with one full pint of water
	BREAKFAST (when we really feel hungry)	Sixteen to thirty-two ounces of the Glowing Green Juice Wait twenty minutes, and only if you are still hungry, follow with a piece of fruit or the Glowing Green Smoothie
	LUNCH	Large bowl of Dharma's Kale Salad Followed by a bowl of Cauliflower Energy Soup
	SNACK (optional at least three hours later)	Eight to twenty ounces of the Glowing Green Smoothie
	DINNER	Start with a digestive enzyme Large serving of green salad with Kim's Classic Dressing Followed by Beauty Nut Pâté or Bruce's Pine Nut Parmesan on collard green wraps
	BEFORE BED	One probiotic supplement Two to four capsules of a magnesium-oxygen supplement, as needed

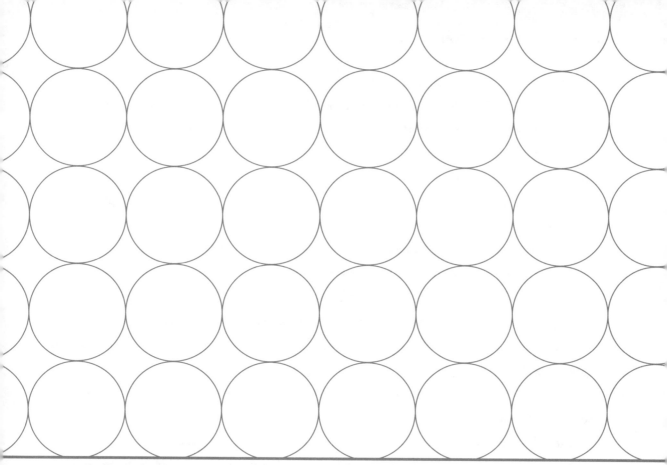

CHAPTER ELEVEN

BEAUTY RECIPES

Nothing will benefit human health and increase the chances for survival of life on Earth as much as the evolution to a vegetarian diet.

—Albert Einstein

When I started making changes in my diet years ago, I was really excited about new and complex recipes. I would spend hours in the kitchen experimenting. Now I truly understand that the more simply we eat, the better it is for digestion. Simplicity is a beautiful thing and will make us more beautiful! If we eat more simply, we will appreciate natural flavors better and our taste buds will stop craving excessively sweet and salty flavors, fancy sauces and dishes with ninety things in them. Food can taste great if it is based on simplicity and natural flavors!

Today I eat very simply myself. I have green drinks during the day and often throw together green salads with Kim's Classic Dressing or make versions of the Ananda Burrito, which could be as basic as a nori wrapper with avocado, sprouts and some spices thrown on top. For dinner I have a huge salad, usually Dharma's Kale Salad, along with some of the grain dishes or nut pâtés I present in this chapter, a few times a week. Sometimes I'll just have a small side of quinoa or millet with my salad, totally plain!

When we come into a new diet, it is natural to feel that we need lots of new recipes to cling to in order to find our way. But that simply is not true! We need to focus on shifting our mind-set to the fact that greens, other vegetables and fruits—the real gifts of nature— should make up the vast majority of our diet. None of us need to spend hours in the kitchen. We can all chop vegetables and fruit, throw them in the blender, and make a Glowing Green Smoothie. We can all learn to make some easy salads, such as the ones I list for you here. These salads should be the *bulk* of lunch and dinner. Salad is not an appetizer or a side dish. It is the main part! You'll notice that the largest subsection of the recipe section is salad dressings. Guess why. To help keep you focused on eating those enormous salads every single day!

We come from a culture that loves to make things seem so complicated—from skin-care routines and zillions of makeup products, to dozens of supplements, over-the-counter medications and chemical remedies stacked on aisles of shelves. This is not useful! The more we embrace the notion that Mother Nature provides us with all that we need, the better off we will be. We don't need processed foods, and we certainly don't need fancy recipes. In fact, the more fancy and complex a recipe is, the greater the possibility that it incorporates poor Beauty Food Pairing.

So here are the simple, nourishing and delicious recipes…which are enough for you to stick to the plan and start getting beautiful and detoxing on a daily basis!

The Everyday Beauty Basics
Glowing Green Smoothie 197
Glowing Green Juice 198
Probiotic & Enzyme Salad 199
Raw Rolled Oat Cereal (for my Blossoming Beauties) 200

Beauty Dips and Dressings
Raw Chickpea-Less Hummus 200
Sally's Salsa 201
Beauty Guacamole 201
Green Bean–Miso Dip 202
Kim's Classic Dressing 202
Dreamy Creamy Avocado Dressing 203
Omega-3 Flax Dressing 204
Sweet Basil-Lime Dressing 204
Asian Miso-Carrot Dressing 204
Oil-Free Red Pepper and Cilantro Dressing 205
Oil-Free/Balsamic-Free Italian Vinaigrette Dressing 205
Oil-Free Basil Lover's Dressing 206
Minty Fresh Salad Dressing 206

Beauty Salads
Dharma's Kale Salad 207
Sunday Salad 208
Raw Tabouli Salad with Hemp Seeds 208
Israeli Chopped Salad 209
Spirulina Spinach Salad 210
Avo-Tomato Lunch Plate 210

Beauty Wraps and Sandwiches
Fresh Romaine Soft Tacos 211
Open-Faced Avo Beauty Sandwich 211
The Ananda Burrito 212

Beauty Soups and Veggie Dishes
Raw Red Pepper and Tomato Soup 213
Cauliflower Energy Soup 213
Delish Squash Bisque 214
East-West Baked Vegetables 215

Basic Yams 215
Italian-Style Sweet Potatoes 216
Ganesha's Sweet Potatoes 216

Beauty Grain Dishes
Millet "Couscous" Salad 217
Veggie-Turmeric Quinoa 218
Rainbow Stuffed Peppers 219
Alkaline-Grain Veggie Burgers 220
Greek-Inspired Millet Salad 221
Quinoa, Avocado and Corn Salad 221

Beauty Nut Dishes
Bruce's Pine Nut Parmesan 222
Beauty Nut Pâté 223
Macadamia Nut and Sundried Tomato Mash 224
The JMP Raw Lasagna 224

Beauty Smoothies
Homemade Almond or Hazelnut Milk 226
Rain Forest Acai Smoothie 227
Thirty-Second Spirulina Superfood Drink 227
Watermelon Slush Smoothie 228

Beauty Desserts
Raw Pecan Love Pie 228
Happy Cow Dairy-Free Hot Chocolate 229
Raw Cacao Truffles 229
Chia Seed Delight 230

THE EVERYDAY BEAUTY BASICS

GLOWING GREEN SMOOTHIE

YIELD: about 60 ounces

All right, my loves, remember that this is the true shining star of the whole plan! Blossoming Beauties, don't worry. You will get to enjoy this soon enough. For everyone else, remember that I encourage you to mix and match seasonal greens and fruit for this smoothie. If you love arugula or kale, throw it in the mix! (The exception is melons, which should always be eaten on their own.)

The Glowing Green Smoothie is best when cold. Here is where a good blender is absolutely critical so it tastes right. See page 161 and my website (www.kimberlysnyder.net) for more info. A good blender is the only new piece of kitchen equipment you'll really need to invest in, but down the line you may decide also to get a juicer. It also tastes best when made with a high quality blender. When made properly, the smoothie won't be chunky at all, but nice and smooth.

Some of us like to throw a few ice cubes in there, which is fine. It keeps okay covered in the fridge for up to two days. For my busy friends, you can make a big batch once a week and freeze it in portion-sized glass containers. You can then thaw out your serving for the next day the night before. This can really help you stick to the plan and ensure you are getting your Glowing Green Smoothie every morning.

Lastly, I'll say to my newbies that you are in for a treat! You would never think a bright green drink would be so delicious…but it is!

INGREDIENTS

1½ cups water

1 head organic romaine lettuce, chopped

½ head of large bunch or ¾ of small bunch organic spinach

3–4 stalks organic celery

1 organic apple, cored and chopped

1 organic pear, cored and chopped

1 organic banana

Juice of ½ organic lemon

Optional:

⅓ bunch organic cilantro (stems okay)

⅓ bunch organic parsley (stems okay)

DIRECTIONS:

Add the water and chopped head of romaine and spinach to the blender. Starting the blender on a low speed, mix until smooth. Gradually moving to higher speeds, add the celery, apple and pear. Add the cilantro and parsley if you choose. Add the banana and lemon juice last.

▶ BEAUTY SECRET

Fresh herbs, like cilantro and parsley, have wonderful cleansing properties and can help extract heavy metals and other toxins out of the body. I encourage you to throw them in if you like the taste!

GLOWING GREEN JUICE

YIELD: about 16 ounces

As with the Glowing Green Smoothie, I fully encourage you to mix and match your greens. But the Glowing Green Juice has less fruit; the juice should be made almost entirely of greens. The apple gives some sweetness, but if you don't need it, leave it out, or if you are concerned about the sugar, you can use stevia to sweeten your juice without any sweet fruit at all. The lemon really helps cut through the "grass" taste and adds a nice balance. Plus we know now that lemon juice is a great liver supporter!

Here is a partial list of some greens I throw in my Glowing Green Juice: lacinato kale, curly kale, cilantro, parsley, spinach, dandelion greens, romaine lettuce, red leaf lettuce, swiss chard and arugula. Occasionally, you can even throw some carrots or beets in there, but they do have a lot of vegetable sugar, so treat them with the same moderation as you would with fruit, so they make up a smaller percentage of the overall juice.

If you are on a tight budget, remember to seek out local farmers, who usually have really good prices on produce. Local farmers also tend to use more sustainable farming practices and less or no pesticides. Romaine lettuce, apples and carrots are usually pretty inexpensive items that we can source!

INGREDIENTS

1 bunch organic kale, or 1 bunch organic spinach

3–4 stalks organic celery

1 small organic apple, cut in quarters

Juice of ½ organic lemon

DIRECTIONS:

Run all the ingredients through a juicer, putting a small amount of produce at a time through the mouth of the juicer. The juice will drain into a container. You can then pour it into a glass to drink. The fiber will be dumped into another container. With a juice, the order we put the produce in doesn't really matter.

Ideally we would drink the juice within about 15 minutes of making it, to ensure the full preservation of its enzymes. Juicing is a different way of processing produce than blending, and our Glowing Green Juice should *not* be stored the way the Glowing Green Smoothie can be for a day or two. However, in a crunch we can cover it and keep it cold, to enjoy a few hours later. This recipe makes about 16 ounces, which is a good quantity of juice to begin with. Over time you can work up to 32 ounces over the course of your morning, until lunch. If it is more convenient for you to make it all at once and store half of it in the fridge for a few hours, as mentioned above, go for it! Even though we may lose a few enzymes, it is worth it to keep you on the plan and keep your mornings light. Plus you'll still be getting so much goodness from the juice in the form of chlorophyll, minerals and more!

PROBIOTIC & ENZYME SALAD

YIELD: about 12 cups

For this recipe, you'll need four 24-ounce or three 32-ounce clean glass jars that have been sterilized by dipping them in water that has been boiled.

BASE INGREDIENTS

1 medium head green cabbage, shredded in a food processor or finely sliced by hand

Leave 6 of the large outer leaves to the side, intact

LIQUID BRINE MIXTURE INGREDIENTS

4 cups water

4 inches gingerroot, peeled and grated

1 Tbs. unpasteurized miso paste

DIRECTIONS:

Place the shredded green cabbage in a large mixing bowl. Blend the Liquid Brine Mixture in your blender until smooth, and pour over the shredded cabbage. Mix very well. Pack the mixture into the sterilized glass jars. Use a wooden spoon to really pack the mixture in tightly. Leave 2 inches of room at the top of the jars so the salad has room to expand. Fold a few of the outer cabbage leaves into very tight rolls, and place them on top of the mixture to fill that 2-inch space. Tightly close the jars.

Leave the jars in your pantry for 5 days. Be sure the room temperature is around 65 to 70 degrees. If it is slightly colder, wrap a towel around each jar and keep in the pantry. After the 5 days, remove the outer cabbage leaves and discard. Move the jars to the refrigerator (which slows down the fermentation process). Bubbling is a good sign that healthy probiotics are teeming.

Unveil your Probiotic & Enzyme Salad and enjoy at least ½ cup at dinner every night, and also at lunch, when possible. Once the seal has been broken on each jar, the salad will keep in the refrigerator for up to 1 month.

BEAUTY SECRET

This is a sacred, super-nutritious salad that has a bounty of enzymes and friendly flora to help us digest our food, restore our pH, increase immunity and make us more clean and balanced. Remember that a lack of friendly intestinal flora is at the root of disease and squashes our beauty.

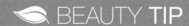 BEAUTY **TIP**

Be sure to buy oat groats!

They look like long, puffy brown rice grains. The pale white flaky oats or steel-cut oats you may be used to using when making hot oatmeal have been processed and are not acceptable. It is very important to get organic oat groats, which reduce any chance of cross-contamination with other crops, such as wheat. For variety, you can replace the oat groats for buckwheat groats, which you must also soak overnight and rinse well.

RAW ROLLED OAT CEREAL

YIELD: 2 servings

I know many of you were disappointed to learn about the beauty-busting properties of refined and packaged cereals, which are largely made out of wheat. But don't worry, because I think you will love how tasty this simple recipe is, and how much the consistency closely resembles regular cooked oatmeal!

This is quite a filling breakfast, and the combination of the fibrous, complex carbs of the oat groats and the raw, fibrous avocado will keep us full for a long while!

INGREDIENTS

½ cup raw organic oat groats, soaked overnight and rinsed well

½ avocado

¼ tsp. Celtic or Himalayan sea salt

½ tsp. stevia

1–2 Tbs. cold filtered water, as needed

DIRECTIONS:

Place the soaked oats in a food processor along with the avocado, and blend. Add the sea salt and stevia. If you like it thick and chunky, you can nix adding the water altogether. Otherwise, you can add 1 tablespoon to make it a bit thinner, and add a second tablespoon as needed. Enjoy after you've had your celery sticks, raw spinach or other veggies first!

BEAUTY DIPS AND DRESSINGS

RAW CHICKPEA-LESS HUMMUS

YIELD: 6–8+ servings

This yummy dip has been a crowd pleaser at many events and parties I've hosted. Because it has a zucchini base instead of a chickpea base, it is lighter and easier to digest. Unsprouted chickpeas can make us gassy and bloated since they contain a mix of protein and starch. I've even been known to use this dip as a salad dressing!

INGREDIENTS

2 organic zucchinis, chopped

¾ cup raw tahini

2 Tbs. nutritional yeast

½ cup fresh lemon juice

3 garlic cloves, chopped

2½ tsp. Celtic sea salt

DIRECTIONS:

Blend all the ingredients in the blender together until smooth.
Dip celery, red peppers and cucumbers in the hummus for a great snack or appetizer.

SALLY'S SALSA

YIELD: large bowl, to serve about 6+

My mother, Sally, is a great cook and was my first nutrition and health guru. I grew up having lots of salad and fruit, and she never gave me dairy milk, soda or candy! I declared myself a vegetarian at age thirteen, and she accepted it and learned to make vegetarian meals for me, as seafood and some chicken were consumed in our household regularly for dinner meals. Besides being incredibly selfless and always putting her personal needs behind her family's needs, she taught me to think on my own and question the prevailing authorities, instead of just accepting information put out into the mainstream as facts. Thanks, Mom. Love ya! This is really her recipe, and I love how she uses bell peppers in salsa. Yummy!

Make a hearty bowl of this every week to keep for you and your family to snack on. It is so yummy. Try dipping veggie sticks in it. It tastes amazing and you will realize you don't need dense snack foods, like nuts. This is the perfect veggie dip snack to keep us on track and prevent us from messing up our Beauty Food Pairings with improper snacks between meals.

INGREDIENTS

4 large tomatoes	1 large yellow bell pepper	2 Tbs. fresh lemon juice
1 large sweet onion	2 cups chopped cilantro	½ tsp. Celtic or Himalayan sea salt
1 large orange bell pepper	½ tsp. ground black pepper	Cayenne pepper, to taste

DIRECTIONS:

Turn on some good music in your kitchen! Then dice the tomatoes, onion and bell peppers and add to a large mixing bowl. Add the chopped cilantro, black pepper, lemon juice, sea salt and cayenne pepper, and adjust the seasonings to taste.

BEAUTY GUACAMOLE

YIELD: about 2 cups, 3–4 servings

INGREDIENTS

3 medium avocados	1 medium garlic clove, chopped very finely	Cayenne pepper, to taste
Juice of ½ a lemon	¼ tsp. Celtic or Himalayan sea salt	1 cup chopped tomatoes

DIRECTIONS:

Slice the avocados lengthwise and remove the pit. Scoop out the green avocado flesh and add to a medium-size mixing bowl. Add the lemon juice and mash the avocados, using a fork. Make it as smooth as you like, or if you like your guacamole chunky, the way I do, then don't mash too much! Add the garlic, sea salt and cayenne pepper and mix well.

Add the chopped tomatoes last, and mix well again. I like putting the tomatoes in as the last ingredient, after everything else has already been thoroughly mixed, because I don't like it when tomatoes get too mushy.

Enjoy the guacamole with veggie sticks as a filling, wonderful afternoon snack! You can also serve the guacamole on top of a large green salad for a great lunch or dinner.

GREEN BEAN–MISO DIP

YIELD: just under 2 cups, 3–4 servings

This is a very light dip that doesn't have concentrated protein like nuts or concentrated fat like avocados. If you like green beans, then this dip has your name written all over it. It's great for an afternoon pick-me-up, sans caffeine, and we won't interfere with our important Light to Heavy eating routine.

INGREDIENTS

¼ cup vegetable broth or plain water, for sautéing

½ cup chopped white onions

1½ cups organic green beans

½ tsp. Celtic or Himalayan sea salt

2 Tbs. fresh lemon juice

2 tsp. organic, unpasteurized miso

2 Tbs. nutritional yeast

⅓ cup parsley, chopped

DIRECTIONS:

Gently cook the onions in the vegetable broth or water for a few moments, on medium heat, until they soften, and then add the green beans. Stir in the salt. Take off the heat, and allow the onions and green beans to cool down for a few minutes.

Add the softened onion and green bean mixture to a blender, and then add in the lemon juice, miso, nutritional yeast and parsley. Blend until smooth.

Serve the dip with your favorite veggie sticks and enjoy as a delicious, easily digestible snack between meals!

KIM'S CLASSIC DRESSING

YIELD: about 2 servings

This is my favorite simple dressing and I use it for many of my salads. There is nothing fancy about it, and I simply shake and pour the ingredients right over a salad, yet it tastes delicious and gives me all the flavor I need—without the need for any oil at all.

This is enough dressing for one head of kale, a container of mixed greens, or a large bowl of baby spinach. I always make the whole head of kale, and if we don't finish it, it holds up pretty great for lunch leftovers the next day!

INGREDIENTS

Juice of 1 Meyer lemon

3–4 Tbs. dulse flakes

¼ cup nutritional yeast

Cayenne pepper to taste

Handful of chopped fresh basil or dill

Splash of Bragg Liquid Aminos or nama shoyu (raw, unpasteurized soy sauce)

DIRECTIONS:

Mix all ingredients together. Throw everything on freshly washed salad greens and toss well!

DREAMY CREAMY AVOCADO DRESSING

YIELD: about one cup

This is an absolutely delicious dressing that requires no oil! Remember avocado contains water and its own enzymes and is much less dense than oil, making it a better fat source.

INGREDIENTS

1 avocado

1 small garlic clove, minced

¼ cup filtered water

1 Tbs. fresh dill

3 drops liquid stevia

½ tsp. Celtic sea salt

2 Tbs. fresh lemon juice

DIRECTIONS:

Cut the avocado in half, peel it and chop the avocado flesh into pieces and put into a blender. Add the rest of the ingredients and blend until creamy and smooth. This dressing can be used as a dip for vegetable sticks or tossed with greens for a fantastic salad.

BEAUTY SECRET

Nutritional yeast can be a lifesaver for those transitioning and maintaining this diet. It gives density and adds a "cheesy" flavor to salads. It is somewhat acid-forming, similarly to how nuts and seeds are, so it fits into the 20 percent acid-forming food part of our Beauty Food Circle. Nutritional yeast is grown on mineral-enriched molasses and is pasteurized at the end of the growth period. As the yeast in it is completely inactive, it is generally considered not to aggravate a candida issue, though if you have a serious case of candida, you may want to hold off on consuming it until you reach the Radiant Beauty phase. It is also wheat-and gluten-free, making it much different than the live baking yeasts most of us think of when we hear the word "yeast," which can continue to grow in our digestive tract and actually use up the store of B vitamins in our body.

Nutritional yeast also contains the trace mineral chromium, also known as the glucose tolerance factor (GTF). This is necessary to regulate blood sugar and is important for diabetics and those that have a tendency toward low blood sugar, making this a very helpful ingredient. Nutritional yeast contains eighteen amino acids and is rich in fifteen different minerals and the B complex vitamins.

As with all new foods that you may never have tried, it is advisable to try a moderate amount to see if any adverse or allergic reaction ensues. For those who don't experience any such reaction, nutritional yeast can be a very helpful, important ingredient! I absolutely love it, and even though it is slightly acid-forming, as I mentioned, I believe the positives far outweigh the negatives, and it has really helped me stick to the plan!

OMEGA-3 FLAX DRESSING

YIELD: about ¼ cup

This simple salad dressing is packed with lots of good stuff! It contains our essential omega-3 fatty acids, cleansing apple cider vinegar and lemon juice, and a bit of mineral-packed sea salt.

INGREDIENTS

2 Tbs. olive oil

4 Tbs. flax oil

1 Tbs. raw apple cider vinegar

1½ Tbs. fresh lemon juice

½ tsp. Celtic or Himalayan sea salt

DIRECTIONS:

Place all the ingredients together in a blender and blend until smooth, or simply whisk in a bowl for about 30 seconds.

SWEET BASIL-LIME DRESSING

YIELD: about ⅓ cup

I love this dressing so much! There is something so happy about the combination of the basil and the lime and the sweet flavor. My favorite way to enjoy it is with mixed greens or arugula.

INGREDIENTS

1 very small garlic clove, or ½ medium-sized garlic clove

2 Tbs. fresh squeezed lime juice

1 cup fresh basil leaves

3 Tbs. olive oil

1 Tbs. water

½ tsp. Celtic sea salt

½ tsp. powdered stevia or 2–3 drops of liquid stevia

DIRECTIONS:

Blend the ingredients together until smooth and serve fresh.

ASIAN MISO-CARROT DRESSING

YIELD: about 1 cup

This delicious Asian-inspired dressing works best on crunchy chopped romaine lettuce. It has a gorgeous orange color!

INGREDIENTS

2 medium carrots, grated

2 Tbs. organic, unpasteurized miso

1 inch gingerroot, peeled and grated

1 Tbs. sesame oil

1 Tbs. grapeseed oil

3 Tbs. fresh lemon juice

3 Tbs. water

DIRECTIONS:

Blend all the ingredients together until smooth. This dressing will remain fairly chunky and thick.

OIL-FREE RED PEPPER AND CILANTRO DRESSING

YIELD: about 1 cup

If you like red pepper, then you are in for a treat. This has a great flavor, so much so that you won't miss the oil.

INGREDIENTS

½ red pepper, seeded and cored

¾ cup fresh cilantro

1 small tomato

1 garlic clove

1½ Tbs. fresh lemon juice

½ tsp. Celtic sea salt

1 Tbs. filtered water

¼ tsp. black pepper

½ tsp. organic, unpasteurized miso paste

1 tsp. raw apple cider vinegar

DIRECTIONS:

Blend all the ingredients together until smooth. Enjoy fresh, or store up to 2 days in the refrigerator.

BEAUTY SECRET

While all peppers are rich in vitamins A, C and K, red peppers are absolutely bursting with these beautifying nutrients! The important antioxidant vitamins A and C help prevent cell damage and premature aging, and also help reduce inflammation. Vitamin K also has great cell-beautifying properties, and helps to protect our cells from oxidative damage.

OIL-FREE/BALSAMIC-FREE ITALIAN VINAIGRETTE DRESSING

YIELD: about ½ cup

The traditional chefs in Italy would probably shake their heads in disbelief at the thought of not using either oil *or* balsamic vinegar in this dressing, but we know why it is beneficial to us to cut back on both! I think you will find this quite tasty, even sans olive oil.

INGREDIENTS

2½ Tbs. raw apple cider vinegar

1 tsp. organic Dijon mustard

½ tsp. Celtic sea salt

1½ tsp. Italian seasoning

½ cup filtered water

DIRECTIONS:

Blend all the ingredients together and enjoy!

BEAUTY SECRET

Balsamic vinegar is acid-forming in our bodies, and we should avoid consuming it regularly. Raw apple cider vinegar, on the other hand, is cleansing and promotes the formation of friendly bacteria in our system.

OIL-FREE BASIL LOVER'S DRESSING

YIELD: about ¾ cup

When I went back to my handwritten recipe notes to type them up for this book, the note I had next to this dressing was simply "Yum." If you love basil the way I do, then I think you'll love this dressing! Fresh herbs are so potent and are bursting with so much flavor that you will realize that you were just conditioned to think that salad dressings have to have oil.

INGREDIENTS

1½ Tbs. apple cider vinegar	½ Tbs. organic, unpasteurized miso	1 cup fresh basil
¼ cup cold filtered water	2 Tbs. fresh lemon juice	2 Tbs. nutritional yeast
3 Tbs. low-sodium tamari	1 garlic clove	3 drops liquid stevia

DIRECTIONS:

Blend all the ingredients together until smooth. This dressing is best served fresh.

MINTY FRESH SALAD DRESSING

YIELD: about ½ cup

This light dressing works especially well on mixed greens. It will leave you feeling super fresh and upbeat!

INGREDIENTS

½ medium cucumber, chopped	¼ cup fresh basil	¼ tsp. Celtic sea salt
½ cup fresh mint leaves	2 Tbs. olive oil	1 Tbs. fresh lemon juice

DIRECTIONS:

Blend all the ingredients together until smooth. This dressing is definitely best served fresh, rather than stored.

BEAUTY SALADS

DHARMA'S KALE SALAD

YIELD: 1–2 servings

I learned a version of this recipe from one of my fellow yoga students at our teacher Dharma's studio. I eat this hearty, delicious salad as the basis of dinner several nights a week at least. It is one of my favorite meal staples. This incredible salad provides a substantial mix of protein-building amino acids, enzymes, minerals (including important ones found in sea vegetables) and antioxidants.

BASE INGREDIENTS

1 head lacinato (dinosaur) kale is best, but curly kale works also

2 handfuls sprouts, any kind you like (I like sunflower sprouts and clover sprouts best.)

3 vine-ripened tomatoes, sliced

1–2 avocados, sliced

1 handful fresh dill, chopped (Optional, but I love the taste it adds to this salad!)

Optional for serving:
Untoasted nori wrappers

DRESSING INGREDIENTS

Juice of 1 or 1½ Meyer lemons (or regular lemons if unavailable)

3–5 Tbs. nutritional yeast

Cayenne pepper to taste

3–5 Tbs. dulse flakes or chopped dulse strips

Pinch of Celtic or Himalayan sea salt

1 Tbs. olive oil (Optional, I usually leave it out.)

DIRECTIONS:

Take the kale stems one by one, and strip the leaves off the thick stems by hand. Save the stems and juice them later. Once you have gotten the leaves off, add a pinch of sea salt to them and tear them into little pieces for easy digestion. It is important not to chop the kale with a knife but rather to use your hands to break it up. Otherwise it is a different salad with a different energy. Using your hands really helps break down and soften the kale, which is important to help digest it well.

Place the kale in a large bowl. Add the dressing ingredients and mix well. Add the sprouts, tomatoes, avocado slices and dill and mix well again. Feel free to add other raw veggies that you love. Cut the nori wrappers (if using) into halves or quarters and scoop the salad into them, making mini wraps. Delicious!

BEAUTY SECRET

Kale is a powerful beauty food that is packed with phytochemicals, fiber and chlorophyll, a major blood builder. The cleaner our blood, the more beautiful we are.

SUNDAY SALAD

YIELD: about 2 servings

There is a beautiful mix of colors in this salad, which I believe truly makes the salad more satisfying and nourishing on so many different levels. And this salad contains our secret ingredient—Cajun spice mix! It adds a great natural kick of flavor. Be sure to get a brand that doesn't contain any salt.

BASE INGREDIENTS

3 cups fresh mesclun or herb salad

2 large handfuls chopped basil

1 cup sliced sundried tomatoes

1–2 ripe avocados, diced

2 handfuls clover sprouts

5–8 radishes, sliced

Kalamata olives (optional)

DRESSING INGREDIENTS

3–5 Tbs. dulse flakes

3–5 Tbs. nutritional yeast

Cayenne pepper to taste

½–2 Tbs. Cajun spice mix (More or less! Start with ½ Tbs. and adjust to taste. I love it, so I personally load it on there!)

Juice of 1—1½ lemons

Olive oil (Totally optional. I usually don't add it.)

DIRECTIONS:

Add the mesclun and the chopped basil to a large bowl, and mix with the ingredients that make up the dressing. Purists might say to mix the dressing ingredients first and add the dressing to the base, but for this salad I like to just throw it all in there! I guess I'm not a purist. Make sure the salad is mixed well, and adjust the seasonings to taste. Add the sundried tomatoes, avocado, sprouts, radishes and olives last, and toss. Kick back, and take your time enjoying every flavor!

> **BEAUTY SECRET**
>
> Lemon is an amazing cleanser with over two hundred enzymes. It is one of the most restorative foods for the liver.

RAW TABOULI SALAD WITH HEMP SEEDS

YIELD: about 2 servings

BASE INGREDIENTS

1 huge bunch curly parsley or Italian flat parsley, or 2 smaller bunches

½ white onion, diced

1 organic tomato, diced

5–6 heaping Tbs. hemp seeds

DRESSING INGREDIENTS

Juice of 1 lemon

1 garlic clove, minced

¼ cup cold-pressed olive oil

½ tsp. Celtic or Himalayan sea salt

DIRECTIONS:

Chop the parsley and place it in a large bowl, along with the onion, tomato and hemp seeds. In a blender, combine the lemon, garlic, olive oil and sea salt, and blend until smooth.

Pour the dressing over the salad and mix well, and you're ready to go!

BEAUTY SECRET

Parsley is rich in the beauty vitamins A and C, and in folic acid, and has flavonoids that act as antioxidants—to put the kibosh on free radicals that damage our cells and can age us. Parsley is also very high in iron, and the high vitamin C content assists the absorption of iron. It is a blood purifier and helps to kill bacteria in the body. Parsley is an excellent restorative digestion remedy. It also helps cleanse the liver of toxins and rejuvenates it!

BEAUTY SECRET

Hemp seeds are 33 percent easily digestible plant protein, and two tablespoons serve up a whopping eleven grams of protein! Loaded with the perfect ratio of omega-3 fats and the beauty minerals magnesium, zinc, iron and phosphorus, these little seeds are perfect little gifts of nutrition from nature.

ISRAELI CHOPPED SALAD

YIELD: about 9 cups

This recipe exemplifies what I mean when I talk about leftovers! This makes a nice big batch for you and your family to enjoy, or for you to have for lunch for a few days. If you do the latter, you could slice up an avocado and put the slices on top for more bulk and it would instantly make a really delicious lunch. This salad is also great to bring to a summer party or potluck.

INGREDIENTS

1 large cucumber, diced (Peeling is optional. I like to keep the skin on organic cucumbers because there is lots of zinc in the skin.)

3 large tomatoes, diced

1 large zucchini, diced

1 cup chopped white onion

1½ cups chopped parsley

3 Tbs. chopped mint

2 Tbs. olive oil

4 Tbs. fresh lemon juice

1 tsp. freshly ground black pepper

1 tsp. Celtic sea salt

DIRECTIONS:

Place the diced cucumber, tomatoes, zucchini and onion in a large bowl. Add the parsley and mint, and mix well. Add the olive oil, lemon juice, black pepper and Celtic sea salt, mix and adjust the seasonings to taste. Enjoy!

SPIRULINA SPINACH SALAD

YIELD: 2 servings

I'll admit it up front. Spirulina powder may be an acquired taste for some. Some like it right off the bat, but some have to try it out for a while before they get to really love it. Remember that over time our taste buds may change! Chlorophyll-rich spirulina is certainly worth trying for the fantastic benefits. You never know. You might fall in love at first bite!

INGREDIENTS

Large bowl baby spinach leaves

1 large tomato, diced

1–2 ripe avocados

2 handfuls adzuki, lentil, or garbanzo (chick pea) bean sprouts, or a combination (to add crunch)

½ tsp. spirulina powder, to start

Splash of olive oil

Celtic or Himalayan sea salt, to taste

DIRECTIONS:

Be sure to wash and dry the spinach very thoroughly. We do not want any soggy spinach for this salad! Add it to a large bowl and toss in the tomato, avocado and sprouts. *Start* with ½ teaspoon of spirulina powder, a splash of olive oil and a bit of salt. If you like what you taste and want to go a bit further, feel free to add more spirulina!

AVO-TOMATO LUNCH PLATE

YIELD: 1 serving

Back to basics, this recipe relies on the flavors of fresh, natural plant foods! Avocado, tomato and basil are a combination that must have made Mother Nature smile to herself, knowing how fantastic it would be when we earthlings discovered it!

INGREDIENTS

1 large tomato or 2 small plum tomatoes

1 medium avocado

Handful of basil leaves

½ Tbs. olive oil (optional)

Black pepper to taste

Celtic sea salt, to taste (optional)

DIRECTIONS:

Cut the tomato into thin slices, and arrange over a plate.

Cut the avocado in half lengthwise using a large, sharp knife, and twist the halves to separate them. Lift out the pit with the knife and spoon out each half from the peel. Carefully slice the avocado into strips.

Place the avocado slices on top of the tomato, and sprinkle the basil leaves over the top. Add the olive oil and seasonings to taste. If you feel you don't need the olive oil or salt, leave them out! I often do. The perfect bite would include a combination of avocado, basil and tomato all together.

BEAUTY WRAPS AND SANDWICHES

FRESH ROMAINE SOFT TACOS

YIELD: about 2 servings

Who says healthy raw snacks and meals have to be time consuming? This is a really fast little dish when you are on the go or Hungry with a capital *H!* It is a great idea to always keep a bag of romaine hearts for this very reason. I used to nibble on a variation of these tacos as a snack when I worked at a raw food longevity center in New York and was taking a break. A few of these tacos also make a great lunch!

INGREDIENTS

1 large avocado

1 Tbs. fresh lemon juice

Cayenne pepper to taste

1 tomato, chopped

½ cucumber, chopped

1 Tbs. chopped sweet white onion

1 heart romaine lettuce

Handful of clover sprouts

DIRECTIONS:

Slice the avocado lengthwise and remove the pit. Scoop out the green avocado flesh and add it to a medium-size mixing bowl. Add the lemon juice and sprinkle some cayenne pepper in there, and mash the avocado up, using a fork. Make it as smooth or as chunky as you like. Add the chopped tomatoes, cucumber and sweet white onion, and mix well.

Chop the hard end of the romaine head off so the leaves fall off intact. Scoop some of the avocado mixture onto each leaf, and top with some of the clover sprouts. Roll up the leaves, and enjoy!

OPEN-FACED AVO BEAUTY SANDWICH

YIELD: 1 sandwich

This is a perfectly Beauty Food Paired sandwich. It is very satisfying and filling, and is excellent as the main course of a heavier lunch or even a casual, quick dinner. It is so much better than all those processed meat sandwiches, which are ill-combined and should be taken off the menu! Typically one Avo Beauty Sandwich is a serving, unless you have been really active.

INGREDIENTS

1 slice gluten-free millet bread or another gluten-free bread

Stone-ground mustard

½ avocado, sliced

2–3 thin tomato slices

Cayenne pepper

Celtic sea salt (optional)

Clover sprouts

Probiotic & Enzyme Salad

DIRECTIONS:

Toast the bread lightly, and then spread on the mustard. Layer the avocado and tomato on top, and sprinkle with cayenne pepper and sea salt to your desired taste. Top with clover sprouts and some Probiotic & Enzyme Salad, and you have a delicious sandwich to enjoy!

THE ANANDA BURRITO

YIELD: about 3 burritos

I have made dozens of versions of this super-easy "burrito" and in fact, it is a lunch food I personally eat often, after a green salad. It is tasty, and instead of using a gluten-filled flour tortilla or a corn tortilla, we are using nori wrappers, which have so many beautifying minerals.

If you bring your lunch to work, you could pack up the filling and the nori wrappers separately, and assemble the burritos there.

DRESSING INGREDIENTS

1 Tbs. organic Dijon mustard

1 tsp. fresh lemon juice

½ tsp. nutritional yeast

Black pepper, to taste

Celtic or Himalayan sea salt, to taste (optional)

BASE MIXTURE INGREDIENTS

1 cup diced celery (about 2 long stalks)

⅓ cup diced white onion

⅓ cup chopped parsley

1 avocado

Untoasted nori wrappers (available at a health market or online)

Sprouts

Optional add-ons:

Handful of baby spinach or a few kale leaves

A few Tbs. Probiotic & Enzyme Salad

DIRECTIONS:

Mix the mustard, lemon juice and nutritional yeast together in a medium bowl and set to the side. Add the celery, onion and parsley to the dressing bowl. Mix everything together very well. Season with black pepper and a little bit of sea salt to suit your taste.

Cut the avocado lengthwise and remove the pit. Scoop out the flesh and cut it in lengthwise strips. Lay a nori wrapper flat on a plate, and lay some avocado strips right down the center (the long way) a few inches from the edges. Next spoon some of the celery mixture on top of the avocado strips. Top with sprouts and any add-ons you like. Wrap up the nori as you would a burrito, by folding the ends up, then rolling. Hold the burrito in your hands so all the folds are held securely in place. Beginners—or anyone really!—should definitely eat these over a plate. Enjoy and experiment to find your own favorite combinations!

BEAUTY SOUPS AND VEGGIE DISHES

RAW RED PEPPER AND TOMATO SOUP

YIELD: about 4 servings

This light soup is filling and can be enjoyed on its own or with a salad.

INGREDIENTS

1 organic red pepper, cored, deseeded and chopped

3 medium-sized, organic, vine-ripened tomatoes

½ organic celery stalk

1 cup unsweetened almond milk

¼ cup chopped sweet onion

1 Tbs. nutritional yeast

¾ tsp. Celtic or Himalayan sea salt

1 very small garlic clove

1 Tbs. fresh lemon juice

DIRECTIONS:

Blend everything until smooth in a blender and serve. This is where the Vitamix is really helpful, as you can make this soup and clean up in less than 5 minutes!

CAULIFLOWER ENERGY SOUP

YIELD: about 4 servings

Cauliflower lovers, you will be in heaven with this soup! I never really considered myself a hard-core cauliflower lover until I started making this delicious soup. Whenever I make it, I slurp it up pretty fast! The turmeric, besides its wonderful health and detoxifying properties, gives the soup a nice yellow hue, so it doesn't come out a pasty white or ugly gray color!

If you are new to raw soups or it is wintertime, you probably won't want to eat this soup super cold right out of the fridge. You can heat it over the stove at the lowest possible temperature, stirring well. Remember that you don't want the temperature to get near 118 degrees, which is the temperature that would destroy the enzymes in this raw soup. So warm very gently and slowly!

BEAUTY SECRET

Turmeric is an Ayurvedic spice that has amazing antioxidant properties. It inhibits oxidation and protects us from free radical damage, and also helps us clean up metabolic waste. It also supports our liver, while adding some bright color to this soup!

INGREDIENTS

1 medium head cauliflower, with outer green leaves removed and chopped into pieces

3 Tbs. organic, unpasteurized miso paste

½ ripe avocado

2 cups filtered water

Juice of 1 lemon

2½ Tbs. of Bragg Liquid Aminos or nama shoyu (raw, unpasteurized soy sauce)

½ tsp. turmeric

Chopped parsley, as a garnish

1 tsp. Himalayan sea salt

DIRECTIONS:

Add all the ingredients to a blender and blend until smooth. If you'd like a thinner texture, try adding a bit more water. Enjoy!

DELISH SQUASH BISQUE

YIELD: about 6 servings

INGREDIENTS

1 medium acorn squash

1 Tbs. coconut oil or vegetable broth

2 garlic cloves, minced

1 large sweet onion, minced

1 tsp. grated ginger

½–1 tsp. Celtic or Himalayan sea salt, or to taste

¼ tsp. black pepper

3 celery stalks, cubed

2–3 carrots, cubed

2 cups water

1 cup unsweetened almond milk

DIRECTIONS:

Cut the acorn squash open, remove the seeds and the peel, and cut the flesh into 1-inch cubes.

Heat the coconut oil or vegetable broth in a large cooking pot. Lightly sauté the garlic, then add the onion and the grated ginger. Do not overcook! Use medium rather than high heat. Add salt and black pepper and stir in.

Add the rest of the vegetables and gently cook over low heat, until they start to soften. Add water and cover, simmering the vegetables for 30 minutes or so, or until tender. Pour the mixture into blender and puree. Add the unsweetened almond milk. Return the soup to the cooking pot and keep on low heat. Serve and enjoy!

EAST-WEST BAKED VEGETABLES

YIELD: about 4 servings

Sometimes baked veggies are so yummy! As long as we are having plenty of raw greens and veggies every day, it is okay to have some baked vegetables in the mix. This dish is especially delicious in wintertime, when we naturally crave warmer foods.

INGREDIENTS

3–4 carrots, peeled and cut into chunks

2 large sweet potatoes, cut into chunks

1 small cauliflower, cut into ½-inch florets

2 large zucchini, cut into 1-inch cubes

5 cups bok choy, chopped into 1-inch pieces

3 Tbs. fresh parsley

1 Tbs. dried rosemary

¼ cup Bragg Liquid Aminos or nama shoyu

¼ cup raw coconut oil

DIRECTIONS:

Preheat oven to 350°F. Place all the vegetables and the rosemary, mixed up, in a glass ovenproof casserole dish with a lid. Add the coconut oil and the Bragg Liquid Aminos or nama shoyu and coat the vegetables.

Cover and bake in the oven for about 55 minutes, or until the vegetables are tender. Add a bit more Bragg Liquid Aminos or nama shoyu to taste, if desired, and serve with a salad.

BASIC YAMS

YIELD: 2–3 servings

INGREDIENTS

2 pounds organic yams

1 Tbs. coconut oil (or to taste)

⅛ tsp. Celtic or Himalayan sea salt

DIRECTIONS:

Preheat oven to 375°F. Wash the yams and cut them into 1½-inch pieces, which is small enough to ensure the yams cook well. Bake in the oven for 1½ hours, or until the outer part of each piece of yam is golden brown.

Top with coconut oil as desired, as well as the salt. Enjoy following or along with a large green salad.

ITALIAN-STYLE SWEET POTATOES

YIELD: about 2–3 servings

INGREDIENTS

2 pounds organic sweet potatoes, cut into 2-inch chunks

2 Tbs. grapeseed oil

1 Tbs. dried oregano

1 Tbs. dried rosemary

Cayenne pepper, to taste (optional)

½ tsp. Celtic or Himalayan sea salt (or to taste)

DIRECTIONS:

Preheat oven to 350°F. Toss the cubed sweet potatoes with the grapeseed oil, oregano, rosemary, cayenne pepper and sea salt in a glass baking dish. Bake in the oven for about 1½ hours, or until cooked through well and crispy on outside. While baking, check occasionally and gently stir as needed.

GANESHA'S SWEET POTATOES

YIELD: about 2–3 servings

A personal favorite! The combination of the sweet potatoes with the coconut oil and Indian spices makes this an especially mouthwatering treat! Whenever I am craving Indian food, I make these sweet potatoes, and my taste buds are completely satisfied. Of course, my tummy is happy that I decided to forgo the cream, heavy oils and copious amounts of table salt that are part of many traditional Indian food dishes.

Leftovers are great to pack for lunch the next day, to top your large green lunch salad!

INGREDIENTS

2 pounds organic sweet potatoes, cut into 2-inch chunks

2 Tbs. coconut oil

1 Tbs. curry

½ tsp. turmeric

1 tsp. Celtic or Himalayan sea salt (or to taste)

DIRECTIONS:

Preheat oven to 350°F. Toss the cubed sweet potatoes with the coconut oil, curry, turmeric and sea salt. Bake in the oven for 1½ hours, or until cooked through well and crispy on outside.

BEAUTY GRAIN DISHES

MILLET "COUSCOUS" SALAD

YIELD: about 6 servings

This makes a great light lunch. Or to add more bulk to a dinner, you can top some of this couscous salad over a green salad. Millet is used to replace bulgur wheat, as it has a similar, harder consistency. We cleverly avoid the gluten by opting for a higher quality alkaline-forming grain, and we won't even miss it!

INGREDIENTS

6 cups water

2 cups dry millet

2 large zucchini, diced

10–12 cherry tomatoes, halved

1 large sweet onion, diced

1–2 cups finely chopped fresh basil (depending on how much you like!)

1 cup finely chopped fresh mint

1½ Tbs. olive oil

1 tsp. Celtic or Himalayan sea salt

¼ tsp. freshly ground black pepper

½ cup fresh lemon juice

DIRECTIONS:

Pre-prep: Be sure to soak the millet overnight in water, and rinse well before using.

In a saucepan over high heat, bring the water to a boil. Reduce the heat, and then add the millet and simmer until the millet has a softer texture, around 15 to 20 minutes. Pour the millet through a strainer and set it to the side to let it cool down.

In a large bowl, combine the zucchini, tomatoes, onions, basil, mint, oil, sea salt, black pepper and lemon juice and mix well. Stir in the millet, and mix again really well. This is meant to be served on the cooler side, so it is a good idea to refrigerate it for an hour or two before serving. Great on salads!

VEGGIE-TURMERIC QUINOA

YIELD: 4 servings

Sometimes you just gotta have some hot food! This dish gives me my Indian food kicks, along with Ganesha's Sweet Potatoes. This is as basic and easy a stir-fry as you'll ever find, and it includes my two favorite Indian spices: curry and turmeric. Thankfully it is possible to get those Indian-style flavors without the cream, table salt and overcooked veggies and legumes that make Indian food so heavy and difficult to digest—and cause all the burping and bloating! I love this dish in the winter. I eat a salad while I'm making the quinoa, then toss the dish together so I can eat it right away, when everything is piping hot. Yummy and satisfying!

INGREDIENTS

1½ cups water

¾ cup dry quinoa

1–2 Tbs. coconut oil

1 medium onion, diced

1½ tsp. Celtic sea salt (or to taste)

1 Tbs. curry

½ tsp. turmeric

1 red bell pepper

2 cups broccoli or cauliflower, cut into little pieces

DIRECTIONS:

Pre-prep: Be sure to soak the quinoa overnight in water, and rinse well before using.

Place the water in a saucepan and bring to a boil. Reduce the heat, add the quinoa and simmer until the water is absorbed and the grains become translucent and soft (about 10 to 15 minutes). Pour the quinoa through a strainer and set it to the side in a bowl.

Heat the coconut oil in a large skillet. Add the diced onions, and lightly sauté for a few minutes, adding the sea salt, curry and turmeric. Add the other vegetables and lightly sauté for 5 to 6 minutes, or until they become softened (but not overcooked). Add the cooked quinoa to the skillet and stir everything together. Adjust the flavoring to how you love it! Some like it with a stronger curry flavor than others!

RAINBOW STUFFED PEPPERS

YIELD: 6 servings

My love of stuffed peppers first started at sleepaway camp when I was ten or eleven years old, as they used to serve them in the mess hall every so often. I used to be so happy on those days! Then, while in my first semester studying abroad in Australia, I lived in a dorm, and the cafeteria there served stuffed peppers often, which I loved. Of course, they always used white rice, and there was cheese involved—not Beauty Detox foods! I like using quinoa in this recipe because it is pretty soft. The quinoa is a good contrast to the peppers, which we won't boil to death, in order to preserve the nutrition, unlike the way that I have had them in the past!

INGREDIENTS

6 red, yellow, orange or green peppers, or a combination

1½ cups water

¾ cup dry quinoa

2–3 Tbs. raw coconut oil

6 garlic cloves

1 medium white onion, chopped

2 cups of broccoli florets

4 cups finely chopped kale

2 medium carrots, diced

1 cup minced basil

2 tsp. Celtic or Himalayan sea salt

¾ tsp. black pepper

1 tsp. oregano

2 Tbs. low-sodium tamari

DIRECTIONS:

Pre-prep: Be sure to soak the quinoa overnight in water and rinse well before using.

Instructions For Preparing The Peppers:

Make an incision at the rounded top of each pepper, about 1 to 1 ½ inches from the stem.

Cut all around the stem in an even circle. Then pull out the stem and the seeds. Discard stem, and save the rest of the pepper top to chop and add to the filling. If necessary, clean out any remaining seeds from inside the pepper and discard.

Place water in a saucepan and bring to a boil. Reduce the heat, add the quinoa and simmer until the water is absorbed and the grains become translucent and soft (about 10 to 15 minutes). Pour the quinoa through a strainer and set it to the side in a bowl.

Sauté the garlic in the coconut oil until gently cooked, then add the onions, and stir until the onions become translucent. Add the broccoli, kale, carrot, chopped pepper tops (from preparing the peppers) and basil, and cook gently for a few minutes. Add the sea salt and other seasonings to the veggie mixture and stir it up! Add the cooked quinoa and mix everything together well.

Adjust the seasonings to your taste. The mixture should taste slightly saltier than your taste, as the seasoning will be less concentrated when we stuff the plain bell peppers. Once you are satisfied with your filling, spoon it into each pepper, right up to the top.

Place the peppers tightly together in a glass baking dish so they remain upright. Bake at 350°F for 45 minutes. Garnish with fresh basil just before serving.

ALKALINE-GRAIN VEGGIE BURGERS

YIELD: about 7 patties

Most commercial veggie burgers you buy in the frozen section of supermarkets are made with processed soy or textured vegetable protein (TVP). We say no thanks to those! These delicious veggie burgers are made instead with actual vegetables (!) and the alkaline-forming grains millet and amaranth.

This makes a delicious dinner. Even my dad likes them, and he has had his share of beef burgers in his day!

INGREDIENTS

1½ cups water	3 cups spinach, finely chopped	1 Tbs. cumin
½ cup dry millet	2 stalks of celery, finely minced	½ tsp. black pepper
2 garlic cloves, finely minced	2 small carrots, peeled and minced	1 cup amaranth flour
2 Tbs. raw coconut oil or grapeseed oil, divided	2 tsp. Celtic or Himalayan sea salt	
1 large onion, finely minced		

DIRECTIONS:

Pre-prep: Be sure to soak the millet in water overnight and rinse thoroughly before using.

In a saucepan over high heat, bring the water to a boil. Reduce the heat, then add the millet and simmer until the millet has cooked to a softer texture, around 15 to 20 minutes. Pour the millet through a strainer and set it to the side to cool down.

Sauté the garlic in enough coconut oil until gently cooked, then add the onions, and stir until the onions become translucent. Add the spinach, celery and carrots and cook gently for a few minutes. Then add the sea salt and other seasonings and stir in. Add the cooked millet and stir well. Adjust the seasonings to your taste. Turn off the heat and add the amaranth flour to the mixture. Stir well until everything starts to bind together and the mixture cools.

Form the cooled mixture into patties with your hands, about 3 to 4 inches in diameter. Place them on a large plate.

Heat a large pan to a fairly high temperature (to prevent sticking), and coat with about 1 tablespoon of coconut oil or grapeseed oil. Sauté each pattie on both sides until firm and browned.

Enjoy! You can put them right on a salad, or if you want them to be more like traditional burgers, cut the patties into thirds and pile them on romaine leaves or wrap in collard greens (see instructions for making a collard green wrap on page 222). Top with clover sprouts, and add some mustard and organic ketchup. Voila! You have a true veggie burger in a veggie "bun"!

GREEK-INSPIRED MILLET SALAD

YIELD: about 6 servings

BASE INGREDIENTS

6 cups water

2 cups dry millet

⅓ cup pitted and chopped Kalamata olives

⅓ cup drained capers

¼ cup minced scallions

DRESSING INGREDIENTS

2 Tbs. fresh lemon juice

1 Tbs. Dijon mustard

1½ tsp. Celtic sea salt

2 Tbs. raw apple cider vinegar

1 Tbs. minced shallot

2 tsp. dried oregano

¼ cup olive oil

DIRECTIONS:

Pre-prep: Be sure to soak the millet overnight in water and rinse well before using.

In a saucepan over high heat, bring the water to a boil. Reduce the heat, then add the millet and simmer until the millet has cooked to a softer texture, around 15 to 20 minutes. Pour the millet through a strainer and set it to the side to cool down.

Blend all the dressing ingredients together until smooth in a blender, or simply add them to a small bowl and whisk well with a fork. Add the millet to a large mixing bowl, then pour the dressing on top, and add the olives, capers and scallions. Mix well and enjoy your delicious meal, which will evoke memories or images of the beautiful Mediterranean part of the world!

QUINOA, AVOCADO AND CORN SALAD

YIELD: about 6 servings

This salad is really great—especially for a summer picnic. My favorite green salad to eat it on top of is spinach.

BASE INGREDIENTS

3 cups water

1½ cups dry quinoa

Raw kernels of 2 ears of organic corn (preferably white, if available), shaved right from the cob

2 avocados, sliced and cut into 1-inch pieces

3 Tbs. finely chopped red onion

DRESSING INGREDIENTS

1 Tbs. fresh lemon juice

1 Tbs. olive oil

2 Tbs. Bragg Liquid Aminos or low-sodium tamari

1 Tbs. brown rice vinegar

DIRECTIONS:

Pre-prep: Be sure to soak the quinoa overnight in water and rinse well before using.

In a saucepan bring the water to a boil. Reduce the heat, add the quinoa and simmer until the water is absorbed and the grains become translucent and soft (about 10 to 15 minutes). Pour the quinoa through a strainer and set it to the side in a bowl.

Blend all the dressing ingredients together in a blender until smooth, or simply add them to a small bowl and whisk well with a fork.

Add the kernels of corn to the quinoa, along with the avocado and chopped onion. Mix well. Pour the dressing on top of the mixture and mix well again. Enjoy this yummy dish with relish!

BEAUTY NUT DISHES

BRUCE'S PINE NUT PARMESAN

YIELD: about 2–3 ounces

I named this delicious dairy-free cheese after my dad, because I don't think he met a cheese he didn't like, and I am always trying to come up with alternatives! I love my dad so much, and he is a very sweet and wonderful man. I want him to be as healthy as possible. Sometimes I even use this cheese as a salad dressing. I also like to put it in those squeezy bottles with a spout that ketchup and mayonnaise are typically served out of, and to squeeze it as a dressing on collard green wraps loaded with lots of sprouts and other veggies. Yummy!

INGREDIENTS

1 cup pine nuts, soaked two hours and rinsed well

½ cup cold filtered water

½ tsp. Celtic or Himalayan sea salt

1 Tbs. chopped onion

3 Tbs. fresh lemon juice

1 tsp. coconut oil

4 drops liquid stevia

1 very small garlic clove

1 Tbs. nutritional yeast

DIRECTIONS:

Blend all the ingredients in a food processor or blender until smooth and store in refrigerator.

Serving Idea: How to Make Collard Green Wrappers

Place a collard green leaf on a plate with the darker side down and the lighter side facing up. Cut off and discard the stem (or save for green drinks!). Add some nut pâté or any filling you are working with, slices of avocado, sprouts, etc., to the middle of the collard green leaf, keeping at least two inches away from all the sides. Fold one of the long sides of the collard green leaf up toward the middle, and then tuck up both of the shorter ends. Then roll the other long side up as well and wrap firmly together. Next turn the stuffed collard green leaf over so the folded side is on the plate, and make a diagonal cut with a very sharp knife toward the center. Voilà! That's it!

BEAUTY NUT PÂTÉ

YIELD: about 1½ cups

This is a very special and delicious nut pâté. It is packed with beauty minerals, amino acids and phyto-nutrients. You will love the taste!

INGREDIENTS

½ cup almonds

½ cup pumpkin seeds

½ cup sunflower seeds

2 Tbs. fresh lemon juice

1½ Tbs. Bragg Liquid Aminos or nama shoyu (raw, unpasteurized soy sauce)

1 small organic zucchini, chopped (about ¾ cup)

1-inch piece of gingerroot, peeled and grated

1 very small garlic clove or ½ medium clove, finely chopped

1 heaping Tbs. chopped white onion

⅛ tsp. cayenne pepper

1 heaping Tbs. nutritional yeast

½ tsp. turmeric

DIRECTIONS:

Pre-prep: Soak the almonds, pumpkin seeds and sunflower seeds overnight and rinse well before using.

Put the lemon juice and Bragg Liquid Aminos or nama shoyu in the blender (or food processor) first. Then add the zucchini, ginger, garlic and onion. Lastly add the cayenne pepper, nutritional yeast and turmeric and blend very well, until smooth.

Add the seeds and nuts once the liquid mixture is smooth, and blend again. You may have to keep pushing the mixture down the sides of the blender to keep it moving, or if you have a Vitamix, be sure to use the mixing pole. If your blender is very weak, you may have to chop the nuts up before adding them to the liquid mixture to ensure that it blends well.

Enjoy by scooping on top of a green salad, but be sure to eat a good majority of the salad first. Or wrap in collard greens with sprouts per the instructions under Bruce's Pine Nut Parmesan.

BEAUTY SECRET

Pumpkin seeds are a major beautifying food, as they are loaded with our beauty minerals zinc, calcium, potassium and magnesium, as well as B vitamins and collagen-repairing vitamin C and vitamin E. Need more benefits? They also contain essential amino acids and omega-3 fatty acids.

MACADAMIA NUT AND SUNDRIED TOMATO MASH

YIELD: about 1 cup

Okay, I'll admit it. This is my favorite nut pâté in the world! I am pretty obsessed with it, so when I make it, I polish it off pretty fast. I made this recipe once on an *E!* segment, and afterward the producers, who hadn't had lunch yet, gobbled it right up. It is particularly fabulous on a bed of baby spinach leaves!

INGREDIENTS

1 cup raw, unsalted macadamia nuts, soaked two hours and rinsed well

2 Tbs. fresh lemon juice

½ cup sundried tomatoes, chopped

¼ tsp. Celtic or Himalayan sea salt

2 Tbs. finely chopped parsley (any variety)

Black pepper to taste

DIRECTIONS:

Place the macadamia nuts in the food processor with the lemon juice, and blend well. Next add the chopped sundried tomatoes and sea salt, and blend again. The mixture will be moist and crumbly but not liquid. Spoon the mixture into a medium bowl, and mix in the chopped parsley.

Enjoy by scooping on top of a green salad (again, spinach is highly recommended!), but be sure to eat a good majority of the greens first. Or wrap in collard greens with sprouts (see instructions on page 222). Right before serving, I like to add some fresh cracked black pepper to the top, which seems to give it an extra bit of spark.

THE JMP RAW LASAGNA

YIELD: 9 x 13 inch lasagna

When we think of lasagna, what do we envision? Layers of white-flour-based pasta noodles sandwiching several different kinds of melted, heated dairy cheese, with some red sauce and most typically some kind of meat. So in other words, the worst Beauty Food Pairing combination you can imagine—starch, dairy and animal protein. And yes, we might also envision the cellulite and flabby arms it gives us!

This recipe is going to change the way you view lasagna forever! There are many varieties of raw lasagna in the raw food community. But I don't want to have to use a dehydrator and wait eight to ten hours for the lasagna to be ready. I am a huge marinara fan, so I think the sauce is really important, and the cheese should taste as much like regular cheese as possible! I think you will *love* this raw lasagna. It is a huge crowd pleaser and will convince your skeptical spouse, parent, sibling or friend that lasagna doesn't have to contain oodles of dairy cheese, processed starch and meat to taste amazingly yummy!

INGREDIENTS

8 organic yellow zucchini

½ cup fresh lemon juice

½ tsp. Celtic or Himalayan sea salt

1 Tbs. Italian seasoning

½ cup chopped fresh basil

3½ cups sundried tomatoes (if you purchase the ones that are dried, you will have to soak for an hour or so)

MARINARA SAUCE

3 large organic tomatoes

½ cup chopped white onion

2 medium garlic cloves

¾ tsp. Celtic or Himalayan sea salt

1 medium garlic clove

2 cups pine nuts

RICOTTA CHEESE

2 Tbs. fresh lemon juice

½ cup water

2 Tbs. Bragg Liquid Aminos

PARMESAN CHEESE

1 cup walnuts, chopped

2 Tbs. nutritional yeast

1 tsp. Italian seasoning

½ tsp. Celtic or Himalayan sea salt

DIRECTIONS:

Pre-prep: Soak the pine nuts and walnuts in water for 2 to 4 hours, and drain and rinse well.

Slice the yellow zucchini very thinly with a sharp knife. If you happen to have a mandoline, you could certainly use that, but it is not necessary. Be careful with your little fingers!

Place the zucchini slices in a large bowl, and add the lemon juice, sea salt and Italian seasoning. Be sure to coat the zucchini , so that every part of the zucchini is marinating in the mixture. The lemon will "cook" the zucchini and soften it up so it has a consistency more like pasta noodles. Set this to the side. Ideally you would let the zucchini marinate on its own for at least 4 to 6 hours before you serve the lasagna. Be sure to mix it every few hours.

Marinara Sauce: Create the marinara sauce by placing the fresh tomatoes in the blender first and blending them with the onion, garlic, sea salt and fresh basil. Add the sundried tomatoes last, after you have blended the rest of the ingredients, since they are of a harder consistency. They will give the sauce a nice thick consistency.

Ricotta Cheese: Make the ricotta cheese in the blender by first adding the lemon juice, water and Bragg Liquid Aminos, then the garlic clove and lastly the pine nuts. Yummy! Don't eat too much when you are scooping it out of the blender!

Parmesan Cheese: To create the Parmesan cheese, add the walnuts to the food processor and grind until fine. Add the nutritional yeast, Italian seasoning and sea salt, and mix well. (You can use a good blender in place of the food processor, but be sure it is completely dry before using.)

To assemble, layer the strips of marinated zucchini in a 9 x 13 inch baking dish, alternating with the marinara sauce and the ricotta cheese. Keep going until you use up all the zucchini, sauce and cheese. Garnish the top of the lasagna with the Parmesan cheese and some fresh basil leaves.

Warm the oven to under 200°F or the lowest setting, for half an hour. Then turn the oven off and open the door to let it cool down for a few minutes. When moderately warm (we want the temperature to stay under 118°F) place the lasagna in the oven and let it "bake" for at least one hour before serving. It's really amazing when the lasagna is slightly warm, rather than super cold right out of the fridge. Enjoy with loved ones!

BEAUTY SMOOTHIES

HOMEMADE ALMOND OR HAZELNUT MILK

YIELD: 2–3 servings

These nut milks keep up to two days in the refrigerator. Unsweetened almond milk can be found at Trader Joe's or your local health store. But there is nothing quite as delicious as freshly made, completely raw and live, preservative-free nut milk made in your own blender.

These nut milks can be enjoyed on their own or as a base in smoothies, such as the Rain Forest Acai Smoothie or the Watermelon Slush Smoothie, or in Happy Cow Dairy-Free Hot Chocolate. These nut milks can also be enjoyed in recipes like Delish Squash Bisque.

INGREDIENTS

2 cups raw almonds or 2 cups raw hazelnuts (soaked overnight)

2½ cups filtered water (feel free to use more or less, depending on how thick you like your milk)

Stevia or dates, to sweeten to your taste (optional, and be sure to get dates with pits and remove them yourself)

DIRECTIONS:

Rinse the soaked nuts very well with a strainer. Place the soaked nuts and the water in a blender and blend on high until smooth. Pour the mixture through a cheesecloth into a separate container. Squeeze all the liquid out of the cloth with your hands, so you get all the milk out, and discard all the nut pulp and nut fiber. If you are in a rush, pour the liquid through a fine strainer (though you won't get every drop of milk out, the way you would with the cheesecloth).

Do a quick rinse of the blender, and put the strained milk back in the blender. Add the stevia or dates to sweeten to your taste, or leave it out altogether if you like your milk plain.

BEAUTY SECRET

Acai berries are loaded with beneficial nutrients and antioxidants, including omega-3 fatty acids, amino acids, minerals, key vitamins and fiber. The omega-3 fatty acids found in acai berries maintain the structure and fluidity of cell membranes, facilitating the inflow of nutrients and the outflow of waste products, promoting youthful, smooth and radiant skin by keeping skin cells hydrated and strong.

RAIN FOREST ACAI SMOOTHIE

YIELD: 1 serving

This doubles as a great snack or a great dessert! I went through a good two-year run of having this for dessert many times a week after dinner! Just be sure to wait at least half an hour after eating to enjoy this, as this would be a liquid dessert. Acai berries can be purchased frozen in health stores and made into smoothies.

INGREDIENTS

3½ ounces frozen acai berries

2 cups unsweetened almond milk

½ Tbs. raw cacao

Stevia to taste

½ avocado (optional, to make the smoothie thicker and more filling)

DIRECTIONS:

Using a good blender, blend the acai berries and almond milk at a low speed until you've broken down the acai berries. Then move to a higher speed. Once it is smooth, add the cacao and the stevia. Add the avocado if you want a denser snack or dessert. Enjoy!

THIRTY-SECOND SPIRULINA SUPERFOOD DRINK

YIELD: 1 serving

INGREDIENTS

1 fresh young coconut, both water and soft inner meat or 2 cups natural, non-artificially sweetened coconut water

1 heaping Tbs. spirulina powder

½ Tbs. raw cacao

Stevia to taste

DIRECTIONS:

Blend all the ingredients together and enjoy immediately.

BEAUTY SECRET

Coconut water is packed with potassium and electrolytes and is especially great when you are active.

BEAUTY SECRET

Spirulina is 67 percent green algae protein, and it also contains omega-3 fatty acids, all the essential amino acids, and B vitamins, and is a plentiful source of minerals, including iron and magnesium.

WATERMELON SLUSH SMOOTHIE

YIELD: 1 serving

INGREDIENTS

1 small watermelon   2½ cups unsweetened almond milk

DIRECTIONS:

Pre-prep: Cut the watermelon into small chunks and freeze 3 cups overnight.

Simply blend the frozen watermelon and the almond milk in a blender. That's it! These two ingredients combine so magically that you won't need any kind of sweetener. But be sure to freeze the watermelon! It is not the same *at all* if you do not. Try it for yourself and enjoy this insanely satisfying summer treat!

BEAUTY SECRET

Seasonal in summer, watermelon has great cooling and hydrating properties, as well as amazing cleansing and detoxifying effects. Always try to purchase organic watermelons that contain their own seeds, the way nature made them.

BEAUTY DESSERTS

RAW PECAN LOVE PIE

YIELD: 1 pie

Pecan pie always conjures up memories of pie being made and given with love. There is something very nurturing and loving about pecan pie! Please note: This dessert is not appropriate for my Blossoming Beauties. Don't worry, though. There are other desserts and smoothies to choose from!

CRUST INGREDIENTS

2½ cups dates (with pits)   1 cup finely ground coconut flakes   1½ cups walnuts (soaked, 4 hours)

DIRECTIONS:

Pit the dates yourself, extracting each pit and discarding it. Add the dates, coconut flakes and walnuts to a food processor and process on high until thoroughly mixed. Press the mixture into the bottom and sides of a round 9" pie plate. Set the pie plate to the side.

FILLING INGREDIENTS

⅔ cup filtered water   1 cup organic Thompson raisins   ⅓ cup maple syrup

1 cup raw pecans, soaked about 15 minutes, plus more to garnish   1 Tbs. vanilla extract   1 tsp. Celtic sea salt

1 tsp. nutmeg

DIRECTIONS:

Blend all the filling ingredients together in a blender until smooth. Pour the filling into the pie shell and garnish with raw pecans. Chill the pie in the freezer overnight or for at least 5 hours before serving. Slice it up and enjoy!

HAPPY COW DAIRY-FREE HOT CHOCOLATE

YIELD: 1 serving

Great for snuggly cold winter nights, or anytime you want a comforting cup of warm hot cocoa!

INGREDIENTS

1 cup Homemade Almond or Hazelnut Milk, or if it's not possible to make it, use a store-bought brand, unsweetened

1 tsp. raw cacao powder

Stevia to taste

DIRECTIONS:

Heat the almond milk in a saucepan, but do not bring it to a boil! Pour the almond milk into a mug, spoon the cacao powder into the mug and mix well. Add some stevia to sweeten the drink, as needed. Kick back and enjoy!

RAW CACAO TRUFFLES

YIELD: about 33 truffles

These are one of my absolute favorite treats—whenever someone tries one, they ask me for the recipe. When I tell them, they can't believe it's raw! My Blossoming Beauties: this dessert is not appropriate for you, but if you get a chocolate craving you can try the Happy Cow Dairy-Free Hot Chocolate or the Chia Seed Delight.

INGREDIENTS

2 cups ground raw almonds

¾ cup raw cacao powder

6 dates, pitted

½ cup raisins

1 Tbs. coconut oil

Pinch of Celtic or Himalayan sea salt

3 Tbs.–¼ cup cold, filtered water

Optional:

1 cup shredded, dried organic unsweetened coconut flakes

3 Tbs. maple syrup

BEAUTY SECRET

In its raw form, cacao contains many beneficial rejuvenating and antiaging elements, including antioxidants and magnesium. It should be eaten in moderation, however, as cacao contains caffeine and theobromine, which is an alkaloid or chemical compound that may be toxic in large doses.

Pre-prep: Soak almonds in water for twenty-four hours, then rinse well. Dry them in a dehydrator, or on the lowest setting of your oven with the door cracked open. We do not want to use soggy or wet almonds in this recipe!

Grind the almonds in a food processor, then add the cacao, dates, raisins, coconut oil and a pinch of sea salt. Once everything is blended well, add the water to make the mixture moist.

Roll up your sleeves, take a small amount of the mixture, and roll balls roughly the size of golf balls, or a touch smaller, between your palms. Add your love! Dip each ball in a smaller bowl containing the coconut flakes, and roll in the flakes to cover each ball evenly.

Keep in fridge to help the truffles harden for at least two hours.

CHIA SEED DELIGHT

YIELD: 1 serving

This is a very filling dessert that helps cap off a meal with something sweet, that will also help keep us from getting hungry late at night.

INGREDIENTS

¼ cup raw, organic chia seeds

1 cup Homemade Almond or Hazelnut Milk, or store-bought, unsweetened

½ Tbs. raw cacao powder

1 tsp. stevia or xylitol to sweeten, or more to taste

DIRECTIONS:

Place chia seeds in a bowl. Blend the almond milk, cacao powder and stevia or xylitol in the blender until well mixed and the desired level of sweetness is reached. Pour over chia seeds and mix well. Let stand for at least 10 minutes before mixing again and serving. Enjoy!

BEAUTY SECRET

Chia seeds are loaded with antioxidants, vitamins, minerals and fiber. They feature a perfect balance of essential fatty acids: 30% of chia seed oil is Omega-3 oil and 40% is Omega-6 oil. Studies also show that eating chia seed slows down our bodies' conversion of carbohydrate calories into simple sugars. This is great for preventing spikes in blood sugar, whether you are diabetic or not. Chia seeds are also highly hydrophilic, capable of absorbing 10 times their weight in water, and of great help in keeping bodies hydrated. Chia seeds gel when wet and, when in our digestive systems, this gel prevents absorption of some of the food (and calories) that we eat. This makes the chia seed a great for those of us looking to lose weight!

CONVERTING TO METRIC

VOLUME MEASUREMENT CONVERSIONS

U.S.	METRIC
¼ teaspoon	1.25 ml
½ teaspoon	2.5 ml
¾ teaspoon	3.75 ml
1 teaspoon	5 ml
1 tablespoon	15 ml
¼ cup	62.5 ml
½ cup	125 ml
¾ cup	187.5 ml
1 cup	250 ml

WEIGHT MEASUREMENT CONVERSIONS

U.S.	METRIC
1 ounce	28.4 g
8 ounces	227.5 g
16 ounces (1 pound)	455 g

COOKING TEMPERATURE CONVERSIONS

Celsius/Centigrade	0°C and 100°C are the melting and boiling points of water and standard to the metric system.
Fahrenheit	Fahrenheit established 0°F as the temperature produced when equal amounts by weight of snow and salt are mixed.

To convert temperatures in Fahrenheit to Celsius, use this formula:

$$C = (F–32) \times 0.5555$$

So, for example, if you are baking at 350°F and want to know

that temperature in Celsius, this would be the calculation:

$$C = (350–32) \times 0.5555 = 176.65°C$$

ENDNOTES

CHAPTER ONE

1. Derek E. Wildman, et al., "Implications of Natural Selection in Shaping 99.4% Nonsynonymous DNA Identity Between Humans and Chimpanzees: Enlarging Genus *Homo*," *Proceedings of the National Academy of Sciences,* May 19, 2003.

2. D. Fossey and A. H. Harcourt, "Feeding ecology of free ranging mountain gorillas (Gorilla gorilla beringei)," in Clutton Brock (Ed.). *Primate Ecology: Studies of Feeding and Ranging Behaviour in Lemurs, Monkeys and Apes.* (London: Academic Press, 1977).

3. R. J. Barnard, "Effects of Life-Style Modification on Serum Lipids," *Archives of Internal Medicine* 151 (1991): 1389–94.

4. Gabriel Cousens, *Conscious Eating* (Berkeley, CA: North Atlantic Books, 2000), 313.

5. Robert O. Young, *The pH Miracle* (New York: Wellness Central, 2002), 25.

6. Lisa James, "Clean and Lean: Helping Your Body Shed Fat-Based Toxins May Make It Easier to Lose Weight," *Energy Times* (June 2010): 16–17.

7. D. Hegsted, "Minimum Protein Requirements of Adults." *American Journal of Clinical Nutrition* 21 (1968): 3520.

8. Food and Nutrition Board, Institute of Medicine, *Dietary Reference Intakes for Energy, Carbohydrate, Fiber, Fat, Fatty Acids, Cholesterol, Protein, and Amino Acids* (Washington, DC: National Academy Press, 2002).

9. John Scharffenberg, *Problems with Meat* (Anaheim, CA: Woodbridge Press, 1982), 90. Cited in John Robbins, *Diet for a New America* (Tiburon, CA and Novato, CA: HJ Kramer Inc. and New World Library, 1987), 184–85.

10. Nathan Pritikin, Quoted in *Vegetarian Times,* issue 43, p. 21.

11. Joel Furhman, M.D., *Eat to Live* (New York: Little, Brown and Company, 2003), 139.

12. R. Doll and R. Peto, "The Causes of Cancer: Quantitative Estimates of Avoidable Risks of Cancer in the United States Today," *Journal of the National Cancer Institute* 66 (1981): 1192–265.

13. Dr. T. C. Campbell, B. Parpia and J. Chen, "A Plant-Enriched Diet and Long-Term Health Particularly in Reference to China," *HortScience* 25, no. 12 (1990): 1512-14.

14. Ibid.

15. International Agency for Cancer Research, "Globocan 2008," **http://globocan.iarc.fr/factsheets/cancers/colorectal.asp**

16. D. Armstrong and R. Doll, "Environmental Factors and Cancer Incidence and Mortality in Different Countries, with Special Reference to Dietary Practices," *International Journal of Cancer* 15 (1975): 617–31.

17. Ibid.

18. S. A. Bingham, N. E. Day, R. Luben, et al., "Dietary Fibre in Food and Protection against Colorectal Cancer in the European Prospective Investigation into Cancer and Nutrition (EPIC); an Observational Study," *Lancet* 361 (2003): 1496–501.

19. Ibid.

20. American Heart Association, "Heart Disease and Stroke Statistics—2010 Update."

21. Ibid.

22. D. Ornish, S. E. Brown, L. W. Scherwitz, et al., "Can Lifestyle Changes Reverse Coronary Heart Disease?" *Lancet* 336 (1990): 129–33.

23. D. Ornish, "Avoiding Revascularization with Lifestyle Changes: The Multicenter Lifestyle Demonstration Project," *American Journal of Cardiology* 82 (1998): 72T–76T.

24. American Diabetes Association, "National Diabetes Fact Sheet, 2007." **http://www.diabetes.org/diabetes-basics/diabetes-statistics**

25. Ibid.

26. J. W. Anderson, "Dietary Fiber in Nutrition Management of Diabetes," in *Dietary Fiber: Basic and Clinical Aspects,* ed. G. V. Vahouny and D. Kritchevsky (New York: Plenum Press, 1986), 343–60.

27. Ibid.

28. Ibid.

29. T. T. Shintani, S. Beckham, A. C. Brown, et al., "The Hawaii Diet: Ad Libitum High Carbohydrate, Low Fat Multi-cultural Diet for the Reduction of Chronic Disease Risk Factors: Obesity, Hypertension, Hypercholesterolemia, and Hyperglycemia," *Hawai'i Medical Journal* 60 (2001): 69–73.

30. M. Hindhede, "The Effect of Food Restrictions During War on Mortality in Copenhagen," *Journal of the American Medical Association* 74, no. 6 (1920): 381.

31. Ibid.

32. A. Strom and R. A. Jensen, "Mortality From Circulatory Diseases in Norway, 1940–1945," *Lancet* 260 (1951): 126–29.

33. Ibid.

34. Vic Sussman, *The Vegetarian Alternative* (Emmaus, PA: Rodale Press, 1978), 55.

35. The Physician's Committee for Responsible Medicine website. **http://www.pcrm.org**

CHAPTER TWO

1. Tom Bohager, *Enzymes: What the Experts Know* (Prescott, AZ: One World Press, 2006), 40.

2. David Jubb and Annie Padden, *Lifefood Recipe Book: Living on Life Force* (Berkeley, CA: North Atlantic Books, 2003), 4.

3. Arnold Ehret, *Mucusless Diet Healing System* (New York: Benedict Lust Publications, 2002), 3.

4. Robert O. Young, Ph.D. *The pH Miracle* (New York: Wellness Central, Hachette Book Group, 2002), 42.

5. Norman W. Walker, *Colon Health* (Prescott, AZ: Norwalk Press, 1979), 3.

6. Young, *The pH Miracle,* 13.

7. Ibid.

8. Jane E. Brody, "Exploring a Low-Acid Diet for Bone Health," *New York Times,* Health section. Published November 23, 2009.

9. Ibid.

10. M. Hegsted, S. A. Schuette, M. B. Zemel, et al., "Urinary Calcium and Calcium Balance in Young Men as Affected by Level of Protein and Phosphorus Intake," *Journal of Nutrition* 111 (1981): 553–62.

11. D. E. Sellmeyer, K. L. Stone, A. Sebastian, et al., "A High Ratio of Dietary Animal to Vegetable Protein Increases the Rate of Bone Loss and the Risk of Fracture in Postmenopausal Women," *American Journal of Clinical Nutrition* 73 (2001): 118–22.

12. Young, *The pH Miracle,* 5–6, 15.

CHAPTER THREE

1. Food and Nutrition Board. "Dietary Reference Intakes Proposed Definition of Dietary Fiber," National Academy of Sciences. Washington, D.C., 2001, 2.

2. John A. McDougall, *Digestive Tune-Up* (Summertown, TN: Healthy Living Publications, 2008), 76.

3. G. R. Howe, "Dietary Intake of Fiber and Decreased Risk of Cancers of the Colon and the Rectum: Evidence from the Combined Analysis of 13 Case-Control Studies," *Journal of the National Cancer Institute* 84, no. 24 (December 1992): 1887–96.

4. McDougall, *Digestive Tune-Up,* 76.

5. Ibid.

6. Department of Health and Human Services. Report on All Adverse Reactions in the Adverse Reaction Monitoring System. February 25 and 28, 1994.

7. W. L. Hall, D. J. Millward, P. J. Rogers and L. M. Morgan, "Physiological Mechanisms Mediating Aspartame-Induced Satiety," *Physiology & Behavior* 78, nos. 4–5 (April 2003): 557–62.

8. L. N. Chen and E. S. Parham, "College Students' Use of High-Intensity Sweeteners is Not Consistently Associated with Sugar Consumption," *Journal of the American Dietetic Association* 91 (1991): 686–90.

9. *Behavioral Neuroscience* 122, no. 1 (February 2008): 161–73.

10. Mohamed B. Abou-Donia, Eman M. El-Masry, Ali A. Abdel-Rahman, Roger E. McLendon and Susan S. Schiffman, "Splenda Alters Gut Microflora and Increases Intestinal P-Glycoprotein and Cytochrome P-450 in Male Rats," *Journal of Toxicology and Environmental Health,* Part A 71, no. 21 (2008): 1415–29.

11. R. F. Kushner et al., "Implementing Nutrition into the Medical Curriculum: A User's Guide," *American Journal of Clinical Nutrition* 52, no. 2 (August 1990): 401–3.

  D. C. Heimburger, V. A. Stallings, and L. Routzahn, "Survey of Clinical Nutrition Training Programs for Physicians," *American Journal of Clinical Nutrition* 68, no. 6 (December 1998): 1174–79.

12. Herbert M. Shelton, *Food Combining Made Easy* (San Antonio, TX: Willow Publishing, 1982), 56.

13. Dr. Ann Wigmore, *The Hippocrates Diet and Health Program* (New York: Avery, 1984).

14. Cited in Harvey Diamond and Marilyn Diamond, *Fit for Life* (New York: Warner Books, 1985), 46–47.

15. The concept of Beauty Food Pairing is based upon the writings and works of Dr. Herbert M. Shelton, Dr. Ann Wigmore, Dr. Norman Walker and Harvey and Marilyn Diamond. Specific books the following information was pulled from include *Food Combining Made Easy,* by Dr. Herbert Shelton, *Become Younger* and *The Vegetarian Guide to Diet & Salad,* by Dr. Norman Walker, *Fit for Life,* by Harvey and Marilyn Diamond, and the *Living Food Lifestyle™ Textbook* from the Ann Wigmore Natural Health Institute in Puerto Rico.

16. Dr. N. W. Walker, *Become Younger* (Summertown, TN: Norwalk Press, 1995).

17. Some fermentation is the result of constructive destruction.

18. Walker, *Become Younger,* 37.

19. Diamond, *Fit for Life,* 51.

20. Shelton, *Food Combining Made Easy,* 36.

21. I give credit to my dear friend Gil Jacob for first coining the term "Light to Heavy."

22. G. A. Leveille, University of Illinois (1972) and G. Pose, P. Fabry and H. A. Katz, Institute Ernahrung, Potsdam, Germany (*Nutritional Abstracts and Reviews* 38:7027, 1968). Cited in *Enzyme Nutrition* by Dr. Edward Howell Avery, 1985.

CHAPTER FOUR

1. Dr. Gary Farr, "Comparing Organic Versus Commercially Grown Foods." Rutgers University Study, New Brunswick, NJ, 2002.

2. Tom Bohager, *Enzymes: What the Experts Know* (Prescott, AZ: One World Press, 2006), 10.

CHAPTER FIVE

1. Dr. T. Colin Campbell and Thomas M. Campbell II, *The China Study: The Most Comprehensive Study of Nutrition Ever Conducted and the Startling Implications for Diet, Weight Loss, and Long-Term Health* (Dallas, TX: Benbella Books, 2006), 30.

2. Patti Weller, *The Power of Nutrient Dense Food: How to Use Food to Feel Great, Lose Weight and Prevent Disease* (El Cajon, CA: Deerpath Publishing Company, 2005), 28.

3. E. C. Westman, W. S. Yancy, J. S. Edman, et al., "Carbohydrate Diet Program," *American Journal of Medicine* 113 (2002): 30–36.

4. R. C. Atkins, *Dr. Atkins' New Diet Revolution* (New York: Avon Books, 1999).

5. J. D. Wright, J. Kennedy-Stephenson, C. Y. Wang, et al., "Trends in Intake of Energy and Macronutrients—United States, 1971–2000." Morbidity and mortality weekly report 53 (February 6, 2004): 80–82.

6. S. A. Bilsborough and T. C. Crowe, "Low-Carbohydrate Diets: What Are the Potential Short- and Long-Term Health Implications?" *Asia Pacific Journal of Clinical Nutrition* 13 (2003): 396–404.

7. Okitani, et al., "Heat Induced Changes in Free Amino Acids on Manufactured Heated Pulps and Pastes from Tomatoes," *The Journal of Food Science* 48 (1983): 1366–67.

8. Cited in Dr. Gabriel Cousens, *Rainbow Green Live-Food Cuisine* (Berkeley, CA: North Atlantic Books, 2003), 56.

9. Winston J. Craig, Ph.D., M.P.H., R.D. and Ann Reed Mangels, Ph.D., R.D., L.D.N., F.A.D.A., "Position of the American Dietetic Association: Vegetarian Diets," *Journal of the American Dietetic Association,* 109, no. 7 (2009): 1267–8.

10. C. Paul Bianchi and Russell Hilf, *Protein Metabolism and Biological Function* (New Brunswick, NJ: Rutgers University Press, 1970).

11. Statement by Margaret Mellon, Ph.D., J.D., director of the UCS Food and Environment Program and coauthor of the report "Hogging It: Estimates of Antimicrobial Abuse in Livestock," given at the press conference announcing the report's release, January 8, 2001. The Union of Concerned Scientists. **http://www.ucsusa.org**

12. USDA Fact Sheet, "Meat and Poultry Labeling Terms," **http://www.fsis.usda.gov**

13. "Egg Carton Labels: A Brief Guide to Labels and Animal Welfare," The Humane Society of the United States. Updated March 2009.

14. **http://www.humanesociety.org/issues/confinement_farm/facts/guide_egg_labels.html** Quoted from interview with CNN that aired on July 25, 2004. Transcript available at **http://www.cok.net/feat/cnn.php**

15. Peter Perl, "The Truth About Turkeys," *Washington Post Magazine* (November 5, 1995).

16. USDA Fact Sheet, "Meat and Poultry Labeling Terms," accessed February 19, 2008.

17. Michael E. Donovan, Official U.S. Department of Agriculture/Food Safety and Inspection Service letter, April 11, 1996.

18. H. Steinfeld, et al., *Livestock's Long Shadow: Environmental Issues and Options* (2006). http://www.fao.org/docrep/010/a0701e/a701e00.htm

19. C. Adams, *Handbook of the Nutritional Value of Foods in Common Units* (New York: Dover Publications, 1986).

20. Dr. Elson Haas, *Staying Healthy with Nutrition: The Complete Guide to Diet & Nutritional Medicine* (Berkeley, CA: Celestial Arts, 2006).

21. A. Costantini, "Etiology and Prevention of Atherosclerosis," Fungalbionics Series. 1998/99.

22. M. C. Lancaster, F. P. Jenkins and J. M. Philip, "Toxicity Associated with Certain Samples of Ground-Nuts," *Nature* 192 (1961): 1095–96.

23. G. N. Wogan and P. M. Newberne, "Dose-Response Characteristics of Aflatoxin B1 Carcinogenesis in the Rat," *Cancer Research* 27 (1967): 2370–76. G. N. Wogan, S. Paglialunga and P. M. Newberne, "Carcinogenic effects of low dietary levels of aflatoxin B1 in rats," *Food and Cosmetics Toxicology* 12 (1974): 681–85.

25. Environment, Health and Safety online. http://www.ehso.com/ehshome/aflatoxin.php

26. Sally Fallon and Mary G. Enig., Ph.D., "Newest Research on Why You Should Avoid Soy," *Nexus Magazine* 7, no. 3 (April–May 2000).

27. Dr. Gabriel Cousens, *Rainbow Green Live-Food Cuisine* (Berkeley, CA: North Atlantic Books, 2003).

28. Joseph J. Rackis, et al., "The USDA Trypsin Inhibitor Study. I. Background, Objectives and Procedural Details," *Qualification of Plant Foods in Human Nutrition* 35 (1985).

29. R. L. Divi, H. C. Chang and D. R. Doerge, "Identification, Characterization and Mechanisms of Anti-Thyroid Activity of Isoflavones from Soybeans," *Biochemical Pharmacology* 54 (1997): 1087–96.

30. Daniel R. Doerge, "Inactivation of Thyroid Peroxidase by Genistein and Daidzein in Vitro and in Vivo; Mechanism for Anti-Thyroid Activity of Soy," presented at the November 1999 Soy Symposium in Washington, DC, National Center for Toxicological Research, Jefferson, AR.

31. Brian Ross and Richard D. Allyn, "The Other Side of Soy," June 9, 2000. http://web.archive.org/web/20000815204236/http://abcnews.go.com/onair/2020/2020_000609_soy_feature.html

32. Ibid.

33. Dr. Joseph Mercola, "Soy is an Endocrine Disrupter and Can Disrupt Your Child's Health." Mercola.com. January 16, 2002.

34. C. Irvine, et al., "The Potential Adverse Effects of Soybean Phytoestrogens in Infant Feeding," *New Zealand Medical Journal* (May 24, 1995): 318.

35. Elisabeth Leamy, "Secrets in Your Food. Genetically Modified Food: Is it Safe?" *Good Morning America.* August 21, 2006. http://abcnews.go.com

36. Ibid.

37. Michael Pollan, *In Defense of Food: An Eater's Manifesto* (New York: Penguin Group, 2008), 23.

38. Campbell, *The China Study,* 6.

39. Harvey Diamond and Marilyn Diamond, *Fit for Life* (New York: Warner Books, 1985), 107.

40. Reichelt KL, Knivsberg A-M, Lind G, Nødland M (1991). "Probable etiology and possible treatment of childhood autism," *Brain Dysfunct* 4: 308–19.

41. J. M. Chan and E. L. Giovannucci, "Dairy Products, Calcium, and Vitamin D and Risk of Prostate Cancer," *Epidemiological Reviews* 23 (2001), 87–92.

42. Campbell, *The China Study,* 6.

43. Robert O. Young, *The pH Miracle* (New York: Wellness Central, 2002), 45.

44. Dr. Joel Fuhrman, *Eat to Live* (New York: Little, Brown and Company, 2003), 84.

45. S. Maggi, J. L. Kelsey, J. Litvak and S. P. Hayes, "Incidence of Hip Fractures in the Elderly: A Cross-National Analysis," *Osteoporosis International* 1: 232–41.

46. B. J. Abelow, T. R. Holford and K. L. Insogna, "Cross-Cultural Association between Dietary Animal Protein and Hip Fracture: A Hypothesis," *Calcified Tissue International* 50 (1992): 14–18.

47. L. Allen, et al., "Protein-Induced Hypercalcuria: A Longer-Term Study," *American Journal of Clinical Nutrition,* 32 (1979): 741.

48. Cited in Joel Furhman, *Eat to Live* (New York: Little, Brown and Company, 2003), 85.

49. Elizabeth J. Parks, Lauren E. Skokan, Maureen T. Timlin and Carlus S. Dingfelder, "Dietary Sugars Stimulate Fatty Acid Synthesis in Adults," *Journal of Nutrition* 138 (June 2008): 1039–46.

50. Miriam E. Bocarsly, Elyse S. Powell, Nicole M. Avena and Bartley G. Hoebel. "High-Fructose Corn Syrup Causes Characteristic of Obesity in Rats: Increased Body Weight, Body Fat and Triglyceride Levels," *Pharmacology Biochemistry and Behavior,* 2010; DOI: 10.1016/j.pbb.2010.02.012.

51. Roger B. McDonald, "Influence of Dietary Sucrose on Biological Aging," *American Journal of Clinical Nutrition* 62 (1995): 284s–293s.

52. Dr. Mercola, "Shocking! This 'Tequila' Sweetener is Far Worse than High Fructose Corn Syrup." March 30, 2010. **www.mercola.com**

53. John Kohler, "The Truth about Agave Syrup: Not as Healthy as You May Think." **www.living-foods.com**

54. L. F. Jackson, "UC IMP Pest Management Guidelines: Small Grains." University of California Division of Agriculture and Natural Resources. January 2002.

55. Dr. Mercola, "Can Low Doses of Allergens Cure the Allergies Themselves?" June 27, 2009. **www.mercola.com**

56. James Braly, M.D. and Ron Hoggan, M.A., *Dangerous Grains: Why Gluten Cereal Grains May Be Hazardous to Your Health* (New York: Avery, 2002).

57. M. Chandalia, A. Garg, D. Lutjoham, et al., "Beneficial Effects of High Dietary Fiber Intake in Patients with Type-2 Diabetes Mellitus," *New England Journal of Medicine* 342, no. 19 (2000): 1392–98.

58. Brian Shilhavy and Marianita Shilhavy, *Virgin Coconut Oil* (West Bend, WI: Tropical Traditions, Inc., 2004).

59. Dr. Gary Farr, "Comparing Organic Versus Commercially Grown Foods." Rutgers University Study, New Brunswick, NJ, 2002.

60. Michael Pollan, *In Defense of Food: An Eater's Manifesto* (New York: Penguin, 2008), 115.

61. Pollan, *In Defense of Food,* 118.

62. Dr. Gabriel Cousens, *Rainbow Green Live-Food Cuisine* (Berkeley, CA: North Atlantic Books, 2003), 68–79.

63. David Steinman, *Diet for a Poisoned Planet: How to Choose Safe Foods for You and Your Family* (New York, NY: Avalon, 2007).

CHAPTER SIX

1. Robert O. Young, *The pH Miracle* (New York: Wellness Central, 2002), 20.

2. Dr. T. Colin Campbell and Thomas M. Campbell II, *The China Study: The Most Comprehensive Study of Nutrition Ever Conducted and the Startling Implication for Diet, Weight Loss, and Long-Term Health* (Dallas, TX: Benbella Books, 2006), 51–67.

3. Joel Fuhrman, *Eat to Live* (New York: Little, Brown and Company, 2003), 20.

4. Claudia Kalb, "When Drugs Do Harm: A New Study Says that Some Medicines, Even if Properly Prescribed, May Kill as Many as 100,000 Americans a Year," *Newsweek* (April 27, 1998).

5. Dr. William G. Crook, *The Yeast Connection and Women's Health* (Jackson, TN: Professional Books, Inc., 2005), 17.

6. Some of the below information was paraphrased from these books: Viktoras Kulvinskas, *Survival into the 21st Century* (Wethersfield, CT: Omangod Press, 1979), 193; and Adina Niemerow, *Super Cleanse* (New York: Harper-Collins, 2008), 70.

7. Humbart Santillo, *Food Enzymes: The Missing Link to Radiant Health* (Prescott, AZ: Hohm Press, 1993).

8. Tom Bohager, *Enzymes: What the Experts Know* (Prescott, AZ: One World Press, 2006), 55.

CHAPTER EIGHT

1. Dr. William G. Crook, *The Yeast Connection and Women's Health* (Jackson, TN: Professional Books, Inc., 2005), 17.

2. Dr. Edward Howell, *Enzyme Nutrition* (New York: Avery, 1985), 142.

ACKNOWLEDGMENTS

This book, and everything that led up its creation, was inspired and supported by many extraordinary people along the way. By God's grace, I am incredibly humbled and grateful to be the channel through which this information can flow to others.

The person who deserves the most thanks, and who I am forever humbly indebted to, is my partner in everything, John P. Thank you so much for your tireless belief in me, and being my ever-patient and loving rock of support as I strive to achieve all my dreams and goals. I love you eternally! I have truly met my match in you. My parents, Bruce and Sally Snyder, deserve an incredible amount of thanks. They are the most amazing and wonderful people I could ever ask for to be my parents. They have given me unlimited and unconditional support and love, even when I have done a few things in my life (like wander around the world for a few years) that some might consider crazy! I love you! Thank you to Auntie Lourdes, who also gave me incredibly warm love and encouragement for my entire life. Also thank you to Poppop, Nana, and beloved Uncle Craig—you inspired and mesmerized me, at age 5, with your travel stories, long bike treks and Asian medicinal studies through Nepal and China. I have always believed that I inherited my insatiable travel bug and wanderlust from you. A huge shout out for my editor at Harlequin, the incredible Ms. Sarah Pelz. If I lined up *every* single editor on the planet and met with each one, I am sure I would not find a more perfect fit for me than Sarah. Sarah, thank you so much for your tireless patience and support for me as I wrote this book, and giving me all the freedom in the world to create my vision. You are incredibly talented and awesome. I absolutely adore you! Thank you also to Deb Brody, Tara Kelly, Margie Miller, Shara Alexander and the rest of my beloved Harlequin family! You guys rock. Thank you for allowing the book to come to life! I also happen to have the best literary agent on the planet—Ms. Hannah Brown Gordon. Hannah, you always believed in me as an author. Thank you so much for your guidance, your perseverance and your friendship. Thank you to Rebecca Searle, my yogi-project manager who helped keep me on track with my schedule and writing deadlines, and was a constant support in believing in my message. Thank you to Curt Altmann, who is a genius designer and dear friend, and who created all the illustrations in my book. Thank you to my favorite photographer in the world, Lenka Drstakova, makeup artist Lindsay Hile and stylist Kent Cummins. I'd like to thank my business partners and team at KS 1Life, which include Rowland, David, Steve, Harry, Tony, Daniel, Curt, Sharon and Brad. I want to thank all my teachers, the Great Ones that came before, as well as friends that have supported me in various ways along my path to write this book, which include (but are not limited to!): Dr. Ann Wigmore, Dr. Norman Walker, Professor Arnold Ehret, Dr. Edward Howell, Dr. Mehmet Oz, Dr. T. Colin Campbell, John Robbins, Dr. Joel Fuhrman, Dr. John Strobeck, Linda Strobeck, Fay, David, Gil Jacob, Sri Dharma Mittra, Dr. Jedediah Wooldridge, Shiva Prasad, talented photographer and dear friend JC Rimbert (and family), Sri Aikalesh, Wesley Adams, Michelle Pelletier, Jimbo Rumpf, Sarah Parker, Maggie Kinnealey, Kari Pricher, Michelle Pulfrey, Maura Mandt, Stacy and Sebastian Wahl, Leila Zimbel, the beautiful and amazing Drew Barrymore, Jeff Lewis, Jillian Barberie, Jon Favreau, Josh Duhamel, Justin Long, Kevin James, Kristen Bell, Olivia Wilde, Owen Wilson, Peter Farrelly, Star Jones, Vince Vaughn, and all of the other celebrity and other clients I have had the honor of working with, my loyal and beloved blog reader family and the thousands of friends I made across the world, from Mongolia to Thailand and beyond, who traveled with me, or took me into their homes and allowed me to be a part of their lives and learn. First, last, and intertwined throughout everything in between, I am eternally and humbly indebted to my beloved guru, Paramahansa Yogananda. Om Namah Shivayah.

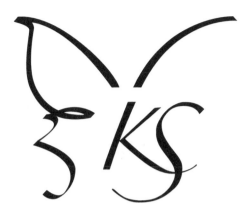

Live the Beauty Detox Lifestyle!

Kimberly Snyder's program and online communities are dedicated to giving you the knowledge and tools to help you live your best life. Our holistic approach provides information on how to improve your inner health, wellness, nutrition and beauty practices—the cornerstones of the Beauty Detox Lifestyle. The result? **A healthy mind, body, spirit and planet.**

On the sites you will discover...

- Products and services recommended by Kimberly
- Breaking news on nutrition and health
- Information on local farmer's markets
- Yoga products and information, including Kimberly's yoga video
- Exclusive contests and giveaways
- New friends in the Beauty Detox community
- Ways to interact directly with Kimberly on her personal blog and social media sites
- Much, much more!!!

Join Kimberly Snyder in Her Online Communities!

Go To: www.KimberlySnyder.net

http://twitter.com/KimsBeautyDetox

http://facebook.com/KimberlySnyderCN

Make this life a beautiful life!
www.KimberlySnyder.net

INDEX

A

acai berries, 69, 117, 226
  Rain Forest, Smoothie, 227
acidity, 5, 7, 12, 22, 23–27, 88–89
acne, 37, 50, 55, 134, 136, 146, 176
adrenal glands, 146
adzuki, 125
agave/agave syrup, 108
aging, 5, 6, 12, 26, 27, 29, 36, 37, 44, 47, 53, 60, 70, 72, 107
  cause of, 17–18
  cross-linking, 5
  rejuvenation, 14, 17, 153
alcohol, 27, 160, 169
alfalfa, 69, 125
alkaline-acid principle, 23–27, 104
  80-20 ratio, 27, 34, 36
  magnesium-oxide, 144
  pH and, 23–24
alkaline foods, 27, 32–33, 36, 78, 104, 110, 153
  eating first, 32–33, 34, 57
Alkaline-Grain Veggie Burgers, 220
allergies (food), 97, 109
almonds, 69, 94
  Beauty Nut Pâté, 223
  Homemade, Milk, 226
  Raw Cacao Truffles, 229–30
  Watermelon Slush Smoothie, 228
amaranth, 110, 111
  Alkaline-Grain Veggie Burgers, 220
amino acids, 84–86, 87, 226, 227
ammonia, 5, 89, 107
amylase, 42, 73, 139, 140
Anderson, James, 11
animal products, 5, 6, 7, 9, 11, 12, 14, 36, 46, 67, 85, 87–89
  acidity, 7, 12, 25, 27, 88–89
  Blossoming Beauty, 153, 169
  broccoli vs. steak, 92–93
  cooking and, 87–88
  in diet, 7, 90–92, 99, 153
  digestion, pairings, and, 45–46, 47

  for dinner, 61–62
  eliminating (limiting), 10, 154, 178, 179
  environmental concerns, 92
  "free-range" label, 91
  meat industry and, 99–100
  portion guidelines, 160
  Radiant Beauty, 154
  rules for eating, 90–92
  sea vs. land animals, 91–92
  toxic body/toxic mind, 93
  True Beauty, 154
Ann Wigmore Natural Health Institute, xvi, 124, 135
antioxidants, 9, 77, 115, 121, 160, 187, 205, 207, 209, 213, 226, 229, 230
apple cider vinegar, 140, 205
  Oil-Free/Balsamic-Free Italian Vinaigrette Dressing, 205
apples, 36, 69, 117, 118, 123, 124
apricots, 112, 117
artichokes (Jerusalem), 68, 121
arugula, 68, 81, 121, 197
aspalathin, 77
asparagus, 68, 86, 121, 158
aspartame, 35
Atkins Diet, 86
avocado, 69, 73, 113–14, 117, 154
  Ananda Burrito, 212
  Avo-Tomato Lunch Plate, 210
  Beauty Guacamole, 201
  Dreamy Creamy, Dressing, 203
  Fresh Romaine Soft Tacos, 211
  Open-Faced Avo Beauty Sandwich, 211
  Quinoa, and Corn Salad, 221
  Sunday Salad, 208

B

balsamic vinegar, 140, 205
bananas, 52, 57, 69, 116, 117
barley, 111
Barnard, Neal, 14
basil, 68
  Oil-Free, Lover's Dressing, 206
  Sunday Salad, 208
  Sweet,-Lime Dressing, 204

beans, 95–96, 111
  sprouts, 121
Beauchamp, Antoine, 135
Beauty Food Circle, 28–29, 153, 203
Beauty Food Pairing, 36–51, 62, 92, 113, 114, 158. See also order of foods
  cheat sheet (summary), 48
  concentrated/non-concentrated foods, 41–42, 114
  how it works, 39–41
  rules for, 41–50
  speed of digestion, 51–53
Beauty Food Plan, xv, 32–63, 75, 99. See also Beauty Phases
  animal protein, rules, 90–92
  beauty food pairing, 36–51
  breakfast, 54–58, 62
  carbohydrates, 105–12
  dinner, 61–63
  fats and oils, 112–17
  fruits, 117–19
  grains, 110–12
  greens/vegetables, 75, 120–24
  "hitting a wall" and, 176
  kitchen equipment, 161–62
  lunch, 58–60, 62
  order of foods, 32–33, 40, 47–48, 51–53, 153, 158
  portion guidelines, 159–60
  protein, 92–99
  shopping list, 163–65
  sprouts, 124–25
  starches, 109–10, 111–112
  tenets for all phases, 178, 187
  transitioning, 150–52
Beauty Phases
  Blossoming Beauty, 153–54, 167–74
  finding your phase, 153
  principles, 157–59
  Radiant Beauty, 154, 175–83
  tenets applicable to all, 178, 187
  transitioning and, 150–52, 155
  True Beauty, 154–55, 185–92
beet greens, 121
beets, 68, 121
berries, 69, 117, 118, 124
beta-carotene, 115

bloating, 21, 37, 39, 43, 53, 142, 144, 153, 168

blood sugar, 11, 13, 32, 60, 106, 112, 160, 203, 230

Blossoming Beauty, 153–54, 167–74

body design, 2–14

bok choy, 68, 104, 121

bone health, 25–26, 70, 87, 103–104

borage seed oil, 114

bowel regularity, xiii, 12, 24, 33, 56, 59, 145

Bragg Liquid Aminos, 98–99, 202, 214, 215, 221, 223, 225

Braly, James, 109

Brazil nuts, 69, 94

breakfast, 33, 53, 54–58, 62
  Blossoming Beauty, 153
  Radiant Beauty, 154
  True Beauty, 154–155

broccoli, 68, 69, 86, 104, 121, 125
  Rainbow Stuffed Peppers, 219
  steak vs., 92–93
  Veggie-Turmeric Quinoa, 218

Brussels sprouts, 68, 86, 121

buckwheat (kasha), 110, 111
  groats, 199

Buddha, 167

Burrito, Ananda, 212

C

cabbage, 68, 86, 121, 125
  Probiotic & Enzyme Salad, 199

cacao, 61, 69, 229
  Happy Cow Dairy-Free Hot Chocolate, 229
  Raw, Truffles, 229–30

cactus (nopales), 104

caffeine, 27, 77

calcium, 9, 25, 70, 103–4, 156, 223

calories, 33–34, 36, 38, 105

Campbell, T. Colin, 8–9, 85, 101, 135

cancer, 8–9, 11, 33, 101, 135

candidiasis (candida), 119, 136, 139, 168, 170

carbohydrates, 43, 44, 47, 52, 105–107, 109–112
  Blossoming Beauty, 169
  glycemic index, 112
  pairing, 42–46
  refined, 106, 153, 157, 178, 187

carrots, 68, 121
  Asian Miso-, Dressing, 204

cashews, 93

cauliflower, 68, 86, 104, 121
  Energy Soup, 213–14
  Veggie-Turmeric Quinoa, 218

celery, 68, 121, 124

cellulase, 140

chard, 68, 121

cherimoyas, 69, 117

cherries, 69, 117

chia seeds, 94, 230
  Delight, 230

chickpeas, 111, 125

China Study, The (Campbell), 9, 85, 101, 135

chives, 121

chlorella, 12, 88, 94–95, 178, 188

chlorophyll, 79, 95, 120, 124, 126, 153, 179, 198, 207, 210

chocolate, dark, 61, 180, 188

cilantro, 68, 197
  Oil-Free Red Pepper and, Dressing, 205
  Sally's Salsa, 201

cleansing, 132–34, 136–37, 154, 159. See also detoxifying

clover, 69, 125

coconut, 69, 94, 227
  oil, xv, 61, 112, 114, 115, 169, 178, 187
  Thirty-Second Spirulina Superfood Drink, 227

collard greens, 68, 104, 121
  wrappers, how to make, 222

Colon Health (Walker), 24

colonics and enemas, 56, 142, 144, 146–47, 159, 176

Conscious Eating (Cousens), 5

constipation, 7, 87, 119, 133, 137, 140, 144, 146

cooked food, 73–75

Corn, Quinoa, Avocado, and, Salad, 221

Cousens, Gabriel, 5

cravings, 35, 56, 57, 77, 109, 110, 142, 171, 176, 180, 186, 188

Crook, William G., 170

cucumber, 68, 69, 104, 117, 124
  Israeli Chopped Salad, 209

Cuisinart food processor, 161

cultured foods, 140–43

currants, 117, 118

D

dairy products, 23, 27, 36, 99–104
  alternatives, 104–5
  eliminating, xv, 99, 104, 153, 157, 169, 178, 187
  goat/sheep products, 104, 105

dandelion greens, 68, 121

Dangerous Grains (Braly and Hoggan), 109

dates, 108, 226, 228

desserts, 61, 171, 180, 188
  recipes, 228–30

detoxifying, 6, 18–20, 22–23, 55–56, 63, 67, 150–52
  cleansing, 132–34, 136–37, 159
  colonics, 56, 144, 146–47, 159

digestive enzymes, 139–40
  eliminative organs, 56, 134
  magnesium-oxide, 143–44
  Probiotic & Enzyme Salad, 140–43
  probiotics and, 137–39
  removing sludge, 159

diabetes, 10–11, 106

Diamond, Harvey and Marilyn, 41

Diet for a Small Planet (Lappé), 86

digestion, 3, 14, 16, 21, 22, 24, 33–34, 36–37, 40–46, 48, 52–53, 60–62, 63, 88–89, 102, 113, 140. See also Beauty Food Pairing
  detoxifying and, 19–20
  duration of, 43–44
  food order and, 51–53
  enzymes for, 42, 70, 73, 113
  fermentation, putrefaction, 44, 48, 52–53, 60, 62, 63, 150
  flora, 117, 142
  green drinks and, 77

dill, 68, 121
dinner, 54, 61–63, 91, 158
    alkaline foods before, 33
    Blossoming Beauty, 169
    pre-dinner salad, 45, 61, 113, 170
    Radiant Beauty, 178
Dostoyevsky, Fyodor, 149
durian, xv, 69, 114

E
eating out, 158
Eat to Live (Fuhrman), 136
edamame, 99
eggplant, 68
eggs, 7, 12, 41, 42, 45, 46, 48, 61, 85, 89, 109, 152, 154, 178, 187
Ehret, Arnold, 18
Einstein, Albert, 193
endive, 68, 121
energy, 16–29, 37, 39–40, 59, 150
    Blossoming Beauty, 153, 168
    dairy products and, 102
    digestion, 16, 21, 37, 53, 63
    food order and, 53, 56
    food pairing and, 38, 39–40, 57
    green drinks and, 75–76, 80, 177
    Radiant Beauty, 177
    True Beauty, 186
Enzyme Nutrition (Howell), 170
enzymes, xvii, 2, 4, 22, 32, 55, 60, 61, 66, 67, 70, 72–81, 94, 208
    digestive, 40, 42, 43, 70, 73, 100
    green drinks and, 75–78
    pasteurization and, 102
    supplement, 112, 139–40, 157, 158
escarole, 68, 121
Esselstyn, Caldwell, 14
evening primrose oil, 114–115
Excalibur brand dehydrator, 162

F
fat, dietary, 73, 112–17, 178, 187
    Blossoming Beauty, 169
    cold-pressed oils, 114–15,

lipase and, 73, 113
    metabolizing, 125–26
    nuts and seeds, 115–16
    pairing, 47, 113
    portion guidelines, 160
    Radiant Beauty, 154
    saturated, 112, 116
    trans fats, 113, 116
    unsaturated, 113
    worst choices to avoid, 116
fennel, 68
fenugreek, 125
fermented products, 98, 160
fertility, 79
fiber, dietary, 9, 11, 13, 32–33, 36, 45, 52, 53, 55, 60, 75, 77–78, 79, 86, 88, 93, 106, 110, 112, 120, 124, 140, 154, 157, 158, 170, 179, 207, 226, 230
figs, 69, 108, 117, 119
filberts, 94
fish, 17, 33, 39, 41, 42, 45, 46, 47, 48, 52–53, 85, 87, 89, 91–92, 96, 99, 100, 109, 113, 114, 152, 154, 158, 160, 178, 187
Fit for Life (Diamond), 41
flaxseed, 113, 157, 159, 171, 188
    Omega-3 Flax Dressing, 204
folic acid, 209
food pairing. See Beauty Food Pairing
food pyramid, 28, 99–100
free radicals, 5, 89, 115, 116
frisée, 68, 121
fruits, 27, 52, 78, 117–19
    best beauty fruits, 117
    Blossoming Beauty, 118, 169, 170
    cleansers for, 123
    dried, 108, 119
    eating first, 47–48, 52, 158
    fermenting, 53
    "fruit challenge," 170
    high mineral-containing, 69
    juice, 53
    lower sugar types, 118
    portion guidelines, 159
    Radiant Beauty, 170, 176
Fuhrman, Joel, 14, 136

G
gassiness, 43, 53, 140, 142, 144, 168
genetically modified food, 97, 98
gingerroot, 69
Glowing Green Juice, 78–80, 154, 186–87
    recipe, 198
Glowing Green Smoothie, 77–78, 80, 89, 154, 176–79
    recipe, 197
glucose tolerance factor, 203
gluten, 109–10, 153
    eliminating, 168, 169, 178, 187
glycemic index (GI), 112
goat's milk/cheese, 105, 154, 158
goji berries, xv, 69, 117
grains, 75, 106, 110–112, 111.
    See also gluten
    Blossoming Beauty, 153
    enzyme supplement and, 112
    four best, 110–11
    portion guidelines, 159
    Radiant Beauty, 154
    recipes, 217–220
    True Beauty, 155
grapefruit, 69, 117, 118
grapes, 69, 117
grazing, 60
Greek-Inspired Millet Salad, 221
green beans, 68, 121
    -Miso Dip, 202
green drinks, 75–80, 157
greens, 27, 67, 68, 92–93, 104, 120–24, 159. See also salads
    best choices, 121
guacamole, 201
guavas, 117

H
hair, xii, xiii, xv, 12, 16, 19, 22, 27, 66, 70, 71, 154, 177
    bringing color back, 146
hazelnuts
    Homemade, Milk, 226
heartburn, 43
heart disease, 7, 9–10
hemp powder/seeds, 12, 69, 88, 94, 209
    Raw Tabouli Salad with, 208
herbs, 68, 77, 146, 197

high fructose corn syrup, 106–7
Hindhede, Mikkel, 13
Hippocrates Health Instute, 41, 124, 135
Hoebel, Bart, 107
Hoggan, Ron, 109
honey, 108, 179
Howell, Edward, 67, 170
Hummus, Chickpea-Less, 200
hunger, 24, 34, 36, 169
    diminishing, 145, 178, 188
    rule, 55, 158
Hurom Slow Juicer, 161

I

In Defense of Food (Pollan), 99, 122
iodine, 125–26
iron, 70, 125, 227
Israeli Chopped Salad, 209

J

juice, 53, 78–81, 119, 120
juicing, 75, 161

K

kale, 68, 72, 81, 86, 104, 121, 195, 207
    Dharma's, Salad, 207
kamut, 125
kasha. *See* buckwheat
kefir, 141
kimberlysnyder.net, xvii, 160, 197, 239
kitchen equipment, 161–62, 197
kiwis, 118
kumquats, 117, 118

L

lactase, 100
lamb's quarters, 121
Lappé, Frances Moore, 86
Lasagna, The JMP Raw, 224–25
lauric acid, 115
leeks, 68, 121
legumes, 95–96
lemons, 69, 117, 118, 208
lentils, 111, 125

lettuce, 121
Light to Heavy. *See* order of foods
limes, 69, 117, 118
    Sweet Basil-, Dressing, 204
lipase, 73, 113, 140
lips, 71
liver, 2, 50, 55, 77
    parsley for, 209
    turmeric for, 213
    water with lemon for, 49, 171, 180, 188
Living Foods Lifestyle, 41
Living Foods Lifestyle™ Textbook (Wigmore), 83
Lobb, Richard, 91
lunch, 33, 34, 54, 58–60, 62
    Blossoming Beauty, 153
    food pairings, 62
    True Beauty, 155
lycopene, 115

M

maca root, 69
macadamia nuts, 69, 94
    and Sundried Tomato Mash, 224
magnesium, 25, 70, 125, 209, 223, 227, 229
    -oxide, 143–44, 157
mangoes, 117
Manipura chakra, 20
maple syrup, 108
Max Planck Institute, 87
McDougall, John, 14
milk. *See* dairy
medication, 136
Mellon, Margaret, 90
melons, 48, 116, 117, 197
metabolism, 25, 54, 60, 61, 70, 97, 115, 125–26, 159
meat. *See* animal products
millet, 110, 111–12, 125, 154
    Alkaline-Grain Veggie Burgers, 220
    "Couscous" Salad, 217
    Greek-Inspired, Salad, 221
minerals, 4, 66, 67, 70, 75–77, 125
    food chart, 68–69
    top beauty minerals, 70
mint, 68
    Fresh Salad Dressing, 206
    Israeli Chopped Salad, 209

miso, 98, 99
    Asian, -Carrot Dressing, 204
    Green Bean-, Dip, 202
mucus, 101–2
mushrooms, 68, 121, 158
mustard greens, 68, 121

N

nails, xiii, 16, 27, 70, 177
nectarines, 117
nicotine, 27
Norman, Philip, 41
Norwalk Juicer, 161
nothofagin, 77
Nut Pâté, Beauty, 223
nuts and seeds, 42, 46, 47, 73, 86, 93–94, 104, 115–16
    best choices, 94
    Blossoming Beauty, 169
    high mineral-containing, 69
    portion guidelines, 160
    recipes, 222–25

O

oat
    groats, 199
    Raw Rolled, Cereal, 200
    sprouts, 125
obesity or excess weight, 6–16, 36, 37, 53
    Blossoming Beauty, 154, 168
    "false fat" and salt, 156
    HFCS and, 107
OceanSolution produce, 123
okra, 68, 121
olive oil, 114, 169
olives, 69, 114
omega-3 fatty acids, 113, 157, 180, 188, 209, 223, 226, 227, 230
    Flax Dressing, 204
omega-6 fatty acids, 113, 230
onions, 68, 121
    Sally's Salsa, 201
oranges, 69, 117
order of foods, 32–33, 40, 47–48, 157
    Light to Heavy, 45, 51–53, 57, 63, 91, 105, 153, 158
organic foods, 90, 121–24
Ornish, Dean, 9–10

P

papayas, 69, 117
parsley, 68, 121, 209
   Raw Tabouli Salad with Hemp
     Seeds, 208
parsnips, 68, 121
pasta, gluten-free, 111
Pasteur, Louis, 135
Pavlov, Ivan, 41
peaches, 117, 124
peanuts, 95
pears, 69, 117, 124
peas, 68, 125
   black-eyed, 111, 125
pecans, 69
   Raw, Love Pie, 228–29
peppers (bell), 68, 121, 124, 205
   Oil-Free Red, and Cilantro
     Dressing, 205
   Rainbow Stuffed, 219
   Raw Red, and Tomato Soup,
     213
   Sally's Salsa, 201
pepsin, 42
persimmons, 117
pH, 23–24
pH Miracle, The (Young), 24, 26
phosphorus, 103–4, 209
phytoestrogens, 97
pineapples, 69
pine nuts, 69, 94
   Bruce's, Parmesan, 222
   "Ricotta" Cheese, 225
plant-based diet, 3–4, 7, 10, 158
   protein, 46, 84–86, 92–96
   protein supplements, 88, 94–95
plums, 69, 117
Pollan, Michael, 99, 122
pomegranates, 69, 117, 118
portion guidelines, 159–60
potassium, 25, 70, 125, 223, 227
potatoes, red jacket, 110
Pritikin Longevity Center, 4, 8, 13
Probiotic & Enzyme Salad,
   140–43, 147, 178,
   recipe, 199
probiotics, xvii, 55, 56, 137–
   39, 141, 199
   supplements, 103, 139, 157

processed foods, 27, 34, 87,
   178, 187
   soy protein isolates, 96–97
protease, 73, 139–40
protein, 12, 25, 42, 44, 46, 87,
   103
   acidity and, 12, 25
   amino acids and, 84–86
   amount daily, 8
   animal, 5, 12, 25, 46, 85, 178,
     188. See also fish
     rules for eating, 90–92
   Blossoming Beauty, 169
   casein and whey, 100–101
   digesting, 42–44, 46
   greens and other vegetables,
     92–93
   for dinner, 61–62
   hemp protein, 12, 88
   high-protein diets,
     danger of 86–90
   legumes and beans, 95–96
   lunch and, 58
   nuts and seeds, 93–94
   pairing, 42–46
   plant, 8, 46, 84–86, 92–99, 209
   plant supplements, 88, 94–95
   soy, 96–99
prunes, 117
ptyalin (salivary amylase), 42
pumpkin seeds, 69, 94, 223
   Beauty Nut Pâté, 223
   oil, 114
purines, 5, 89

Q

quinoa, 75, 110, 111, 154
   Avocado and Corn Salad, 221
   Rainbow Stuffed Peppers, 219
   Veggie-Turmeric, 218

R

Radiant Beauty, 154, 170, 175–83
   how long to be in phase, 179
   sample menu, 179–83
radicchio, 68
radishes, 68, 69, 121, 125
raisins, 117, 124
raw foods, 37, 38, 39, 53, 56,
   73–74, 75, 133, 150, 152,
   157, 162
rBGH, 102
rice, 111, 112

romaine lettuce, 68, 104, 121
   Fresh, Soft Tacos, 211
roots, 69
rutabaga, 68
rye, 111

S

salad dressing recipes, 202–206,
   208, 212, 221
salads, 45, 52, 53, 61, 158
   apple cider vinegar for, 140
   Blossoming Beauty, 169, 170
   eating daily, 92, 120
   eating first, 32, 33, 34, 52, 53,
     73–74, 92, 157, 158
   eating out and, 158
   flaxseeds for, 113, 159, 171,
     180, 188
   as meal, 114, 141
   oil-free, 113
   pairing, 46, 47, 48, 92, 114
   predinner, 45, 61, 113, 170
   recipes, 207–10, 217, 221
   sea vegetables for, 125–26, 156
   sprouts for, 125
   Sunday, 208
   for transitioning, 155
Salsa, Sally's, 201
salt, 126, 156, 169, 178, 187
sandwiches and wraps, recipes,
   211–12
Satchidananda, Sri Swami, 185
Saunders, Kerrie, 14
scallions, 121
Scharffenberg, John, 8
sea vegetables, 68, 104, 125–26,
   156
senna and cascara, 146
sesame seeds, 69, 94, 104, 125
shallots, 121
Shaw, George Bernard, 65
Shelton, Herbert M., 40
Shilhavy, Brian and Marianita, 115
shopping list, 163–65
silicon, 70
skin, xiii, xv, xvi, 16, 19, 22, 27,
   37, 38, 50, 56, 70, 71, 80,
   89, 107, 138, 154, 177
   nasolabial lines, 12, 19, 138
   Radiant Beauty, 154, 177
   True Beauty, 186
smoothie recipes, 226–28

snacks, 54, 61, 169, 178, 188

soba noodles, 111

soda, 26, 27

soup recipes, 213–14

soy protein/products, 96–99, 169, 178, 187

spinach, 68, 86, 104, 121, 124
    Spirulina, Salad, 210

spirulina, 94–95, 227
    Spinach Salad, 210
    Thirty-Second, Superfood Drink, 227

Splenda, 35

sprouts, 27, 69, 124–25

squash, 68, 86, 110, 111, 124
    Delish, Bisque, 214

stevia, 35, 61, 108, 226

sugar, 27, 87, 106–7, 153

sunflower seeds, 69, 94
    Beauty Nut Pâté, 223
    oil, 115
    sprouts, 69, 125

sweeteners. See also sugar
    agave/agave syrup, 108
    artificial, 27, 35, 169, 178, 187
    recommended, 35, 61, 108, 226

sweet potatoes, 68, 110, 111
    Ganesha's, 215
    Italian-Style, 215

Swiss chard, 68, 121

T

Tacos, Fresh Romaine Soft, 211

tangerines, 69, 117

tea, 77, 180

thyroid gland, 97, 115, 125–26

tomatoes, 68, 117
    Avo-, Lunch Plate, 210
    Israeli Chopped Salad, 209
    The JMP Raw Lasagna, 224–25
    Macadamia Nut and Sundried, Mash, 224
    Marinara Sauce, 224–25
    Raw Red Pepper and, Soup, 213
    Sally's Salsa, 201

toxins, 5, 6, 20, 22, 26, 146
    in dairy, 102
    environmental, 92, 95, 98, 109, 123
    as internal sludge, 17–18, 132,

134, 136–37, 146–47, 153, 159
    transitioning, 150–52

triglycerides, 115

triticale, 125

True Beauty, 154–55, 185–92
    basic tenets, 186–87
    sample menu, 188–92

trypsin, 97

turmeric, xv–xvi, 69, 213
    Veggie-, Quinoa, 218

turnip greens, 104

turnips, 68, 121

Two-Speed Breville Juicer, 161

U

uric acid, 2, 4, 5, 89

V

vegetables, 27, 104, 120–24
    best choices, 121
    cleansers for, 123
    East-West Baked, 215
    high mineral-containing, 68
    as neutral in food pairing, 46
    portion guidelines, 159
    raw, cultured, 140–43
    raw vs. cooked, 75, 120
    recipes, 215–16
    starchy, best choices, 110, 111

vegetarian/vegan diet, 13, 84, 87, 88, 92–96, 193
    strongest animals and, 5, 59, 85
    transitioning, 151

Virgin Coconut Oil (Shilhavy), 115

vitamins
    A, 115, 125, 205, 209
    B_6, 125
    B_{12}, 157
    B complex, 124, 223, 227
    C, 115, 124, 125, 205, 209, 223
    D, 70, 157
    D_3, 157
    E, 115, 124, 125, 223
    K, 124, 205
    supplement, 157

Vitamix blender, 161

W

Walker, Norman, 1, 24, 41, 43, 44, 78, 113, 131

walnuts, 69, 94
    "Parmesan" Cheese, 225

water, 49
    lemon with, 49, 171, 180, 188

watercress, 68, 121, 125

watermelon, 117
    Slush Smoothie, 228

weight loss, 4, 6, 21, 26, 35, 38, 70, 73, 104, 113, 145
    Blossoming Beauty, 153
    chia seeds for, 230
    food pairing and, 39, 40, 47
    green drinks and, 76, 80
    plateaus, 176
    Radiant Beauty, 154, 177
    True Beauty, 186

Weil, Andrew, 14

Western medicine, 135

wheatgrass, 68, 121

Wigmore, Ann, 41, 53, 67, 77, 78, 83, 124, 141, 146

X

xylitol, 35, 108

Y

yams, 68, 110, 111
    Basic, recipe, 215

yeast, nutritional, 203

Yeast Connection and Women's Health, The (Crook), 170

yeasts and fungus, 24, 50, 118, 119, 168, 170

yoga, xv, 134

Yogananda, Paramahansa, 31, 175

yogurt, xiii, 9, 41, 99, 100, 102, 103, 105, 141

Young, Robert O., 5–6, 24, 26, 135

Yukteswar, Swami Sri, 15

Z

zinc, 70, 209, 223

zucchini, 68
    Israeli Chopped Salad, 209
    The JMP Raw Lasagna, 224–25
    Millet "Couscous" Salad, 217
    Raw Chickpea-Less Hummus, 200

ABOUT THE AUTHOR

After graduating magna cum laude from Georgetown University, Kimberly Snyder didn't choose an ordinary path. Instead, she embarked on a three-year solo journey spanning over 50 countries and six continents wherein she studied the health and beauty practices of numerous local cultures around the world. It was during this life-changing sabbatical that she discovered her calling in life: to be of service by helping others improve their lives through nutrition.

Snyder is a clinical nutritionist (CN) and a member of the National Association of Nutrition Professionals and the American Association of Nutrition Consultants.

Snyder is the nutritionist for many of the entertainment industry's top celebrities and has worked with clients on some of Hollywood's biggest film sets. She has also been a guest and nutritional expert on many top national television programs, including the *Today* show, *Good Morning America, Access Hollywood, EXTRA, E!, Fox & Friends, Good Day LA, Fox News* and *Better TV*. She has also been featured in, or served as a contributor to, publications such as *InStyle, Lucky, Elle, USA Today, People, People Style Watch, Redbook, Marie Claire, Health, Real Simple, Nylon, Women's Health, Prevention, Better Homes and Gardens, Us Weekly, OK! Magazine, InTouch* and *Star* magazine.

In her spare time, Snyder can usually be found teaching or practicing yoga. Still a traveler at heart, Snyder continues to explore the world whenever possible and splits her time between New York City and Los Angeles.

Visit Kimberly at her website and blog, at www.kimberlysnyder.net.